HD
rge
Print

Shedding Years

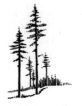

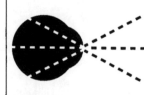

This Large Print Book carries the
Seal of Approval of N.A.V.H.

Shedding Years

Growing Older, Feeling Younger

PHYLLIS GREENE

Thorndike Press • Waterville, Maine

Published in 2003 by arrangement with Random House, Inc.

Thorndike Press® Large Print Senior Lifestyles Series.

The tree indicium is a trademark of Thorndike Press.

The text of this Large Print edition is unabridged.
Other aspects of the book may vary from the original edition.

Set in 16 pt. Plantin by Minnie B. Raven.

Printed in the United States on permanent paper.

Library of Congress Cataloging-in-Publication Data

Greene, Phyllis.
    Shedding years : growing older, feeling younger /
Phyllis Greene.
        p. cm.
    ISBN 0-7862-5586-2 (lg. print : hc : alk. paper)
    1. Aged women — United States — Attitudes — Case
studies.   2. Aged women — United States — Biography.
3. Aging — United States — Psychological aspects — Case
studies.   4. Old age — United States — Psychological
aspects — Case studies.   5. Youthfulness — United States
— Psychological aspects — Case studies.
6. Self-actualization (Psychology) in old age —
United States — Case studies.   I. Title.
HQ1064.U5G74 2003
    305.26—dc21   2003050776

As the Founder/CEO of NAVH, the only national health agency solely devoted to those who, although not totally blind, have an eye disease which could lead to serious visual impairment, I am pleased to recognize Thorndike Press as one of the leading publishers in the large print field.

Founded in 1954 in San Francisco to prepare large print textbooks for partially seeing children, NAVH became the pioneer and standard setting agency in the preparation of large type.

Today, those publishers who meet our standards carry the prestigious "Seal of Approval" indicating high quality large print. We are delighted that Thorndike Press is one of the publishers whose titles meet these standards. We are also pleased to recognize the significant contribution Thorndike Press is making in this important and growing field.

Lorraine H. Marchi, L.H.D.
Founder/CEO
NAVH

Acknowledgments

I shall be forever grateful to the people who believed that I could begin a writing career just as I reached age eighty. As I showed my children, Bob, Debby (DG) and Tim, the first snippets of what I hoped could be a book, they asked (told) me to write more. When I had more, Eric Simonoff at Janklow and Nesbitt echoed their advice: Write more. When Villard bought it, Bruce Tracy said, once again, write more. And once the writing was done, I was offered all kinds of support from the caring people at Random House: Brian McLendon, Katie Zug, Janet Wygal, Carole Lowenstein, and the countless others who lent their expertise without my ever meeting them. Without all of them cheering me on, *It Must Have Been Moonglow* and *Shedding Years* would have remained ideas floating somewhere in my mind. I wish I hadn't been such a late bloomer!

Thank you, thank you to the readers who sent me such an overwhelming volume of e-mail and snail mail, sharing their reflections on widowhood, especially the following people for their gracious willingness to allow me to include their stories within this book: Jennifer Wheeler, Margot Bongers, Jean Crawford, Doreen Gray, Helen Baguskas, Jerilyn Mhoon, Mary Alice Rauber, Joan M. Dickert, Cathy Flanagan Mowder, Elnora Koenig, Bella Feldmar, Betty Thompson, Phyllis J. Williams, Marty Vallery, and Nancy L. Lund.

Contents

Introduction

When I was eighty, I wrote a book called *It Must Have Been Moonglow: Reflections on the First Years of Widowhood*, and began to shed years. I shed them in the writing; I shed them in the many responses I received; I shed them as I went on book tours and met my readers of like mind and like age. I got younger sitting at my computer. I got younger walking to the mailbox. I got younger waiting in airports! After six months, I was feeling downright giddy — if not exactly girlish.

I still look the same — with the same wrinkles, with more white in my gray hair — and I'm still sometimes a little unsteady on my feet. But I don't feel the same. I feel good, stimulated, and rewarded. Young.

I had a funny comeuppance when a young Wellesley woman e-mailed a friend that she had heard the Wellesley motto — *Non Ministrari sed Ministrare* — coming from her TV set as she was paying scant attention to the *Today* show. She looked up, she said, to see "a cuter than cute little

11

old lady who had written a book." Cute, no. More short than little, I think. Old, definitely not! But, she was right: I had written a book.

My life is in reverse, and the iMac is the fountain of youth. For me, it is the antiaging formula that beats retinol and collagen and Rogaine. (I would suspect it beats Viagra, too.)

There was a time when I might have been too superstitious to confess to this miracle. I do so now with joy and the knowledge that Edith Wharton had it about right when she said,

"In spite of illness, in spite even of the archenemy, sorrow, one can remain alive long past the usual date of disintegration if one is unafraid of change, insatiable in intellectual curiosity, interested in big things, and happy in small ways."

A Backward Glance, Scribner 1934

Shedding Years

The President of the United States has asked me to get on with the business of living. It is something I have been asking of myself as well; so, at least, we are in political agreement on that score. I am, ideologically, so far to his left that I am not even in the same room with him; but I am, indeed, in the same country. I have been with him since the World Trade Center disaster, and I salute him. So often we have heard members of the clergy say, ". . . and pray for our president," and I have not even really heard the words. On the six-month anniversary of that terrible day of 9/11, as I was falling asleep, I thought of the tremendous burden that is with George W. Bush daily, hourly, every minute — the responsibility for all of us in this world of turmoil — and I did pray for him, in a very personal way.

With a long history of being a cooperative person, I want to do as the president asks. It's the "getting on" part that I am still unsure about. Since publishing *It Must Have Been Moonglow*, however, I have received some remarkable advice from readers whose courage, stamina, and empathy have pointed me in the direction of another book. What their correspondence has done for me has helped me shed years. I am younger at eighty-two than I was at eighty. If putting my life on paper and making friends in the process is rejuvenating, then I see a large investment in ink-jet printer refills, and much to write before I sleep.

One evening at a dinner table, I heard about a woman who, at age sixty-five, decided that she was simply going to stop counting birthdays ahead and would count them backward. Thus, when she turned sixty-six she chose, instead, to be sixty-four. She started back down. She kept this up for a number of years, calculating her age in her own unique way, not only to her friends and acquaintances, but to the bureau of motor vehicles. With each change of age, she changed her hair color, too. How long this went on, how well she got away with it — whether it is a slightly exaggerated story — I am not sure. But it shows a pretty good attitude.

For some reason, I remember being forty-two as the best age to be. When I stop to examine why that is the year I choose, it must be that my children were fourteen, twelve, and eight; I was no longer wrapped up in domestic dailiness and could find a place for myself in the greater community; my husband knew where he was in his career and where he was going; life's problems were present, but they were solvable. So now that I am eighty-two, and if the counting-back theory from sixty-five can work, I'll be ninety-seven when I turn forty-two. There are worse goals to have.

I had an aunt who was so full of love that it spilled out of her — to old friends everywhere, to friends she had just met, to relatives with whom she corresponded voluminously, and, most especially, to her sister's firstborn: me. And to my children. She remembered each and every birthday by telling each child, whatever birthday it was, that they had reached the best age that anyone could be: two, ten, fifteen, thirty. Just reach that year and it will be a wonderful year. When I turned eighty, I missed her especially. Would she think that was the best year? "Yes," I can tell her. "Yes, in many ways."

I feel liberated to be at a point in my life when I know I am beyond changing what has been. For good or bad, I have done

15

what I have done, have chosen whatever I chose, have lived how I have lived. (Of course, I still have to do my best until 2016, when I celebrate that forty-second birthday!) That is a freeing feeling. We do not have to dwell on the past. It is too late for "what ifs." We can be thankful for who we have become, whoever we are; know that we have made the journey the best way we knew how; forget the stumbles; and continue to turn the wheel of our life.

Loneliness Is Not Just for Widows Anymore

In the general miasma of sadness that lies over the country, loneliness is not confined only to widows and widowers; and yet, to each widow or widower there is a specific trigger that evokes a special sadness, as I have learned from the readers of *It Must Have Been Moonglow*.

In the months after the book appeared, hundreds of poignant e-mails and snail mails arrived. On so many days, I wept as I read of courageous caretaking, of utter and abject despair, of a desire to cope so as not to burden the children, of struggles to find grief relief. Every person who wrote seemed to find some small comfort in knowing that there are so many of us on this journey together.

What I heard most often was that we were GeorgeandLouise or JackandMolly or BillandMary. There must be many American Bobs; I heard from JoanandBob and MarthaandBob and EricaandBob. A lot of widows were missing their Bobs; maybe they felt particularly compelled to write me because they knew how much I was missing mine.

The most frequent comment was, "You made me feel so normal." Or variations: "You must have been living in my house" or "living in my mind"; or "wow, it sounds like my life" and "I could almost write a similar book. It would be titled *Stardust*." I'm glad they didn't: these correspondents are so articulate and eloquent that they could well have been published before I even thought about making a book from my journal maunderings!

The far-fetched details of my life have happened to so many others: I expected that a lot of lonely, single people had bought one baking potato, but never did I imagine that at least three women had also been stuck with an unforgiving car lease and had continued to drive their husbands' cars, which were often too big for them. One widow wrote that I had given her the courage to do it. (I didn't drive that big Cadillac until the lease ran out because I was brave; I did it because I was so angry.) This particular letter writer said she just got in her old, small, kind-of-rattly car, drove to her son's house, left the car, asked him to take her home, and got into the more luxurious, newer car and took a drive. She knew, all along, she says, that her husband had understood that his days for driving were going to be few, that he really had gotten it for her so she'd be safer on the road. Courage, I think, was another word for acceptance — for reality.

Just today, I had to fill out a form for my health insurer about the working aged. (That seems to be an accurate description of who I am at the moment.) Once again, there was the awful question: married (check here); single (check here). One woman wrote that the first time she had to complete such a questionnaire in a doctor's office, she marked single and put "widow" in parentheses. And, she added, "I think that actually covers most of my life nowadays. A life in parentheses." Widow after widow after widow volunteered that she hated the word "widow."

I often told these wonderful, evocative stories when I spoke at book signings. The interested, responsive audiences tend to run together in my mind — was it Tampa, Florida, or Dayton, Ohio, or Madison, Connecticut? Yet the people who spoke to me or wrote to me stand out so clearly that I can see the faces, I can see the handwriting.

I heard from more than a few young people who, glimpsing widowhood, were made aware of their luck to be looking ahead to happy married lives.

So many, many devoted children wanted to learn how to help a grieving parent; a twenty-one-year-old girl wanted to know what she could do for her grandmother. The book seemed to be an eye-opener for many young people who had come across it unexpectedly; each one who wrote felt he or she had learned some kind of life's lesson. That was humbling and very rewarding.

It was in Sarasota that a teenage boy was the last in line to have his book signed. He told me it was for his mother, asked that I autograph it for her, and told me her name. When I asked if he had recently lost his dad, he said he had and that, when he read about this event in the paper, he came because he thought the book might help her. The lump in my throat gets bigger; it is hard to swallow.

A daughter told me about her mother who had died suddenly, at eighty-eight, after eighteen years of widowhood. Her daughters had been supportive and loving, realizing that her life was lonely but that she was "coping." After she died, they found a list their mother had kept of things to be happy about! That's a legacy.

It seems to be — it is — universal to have to produce the death certificate to prove that your husband is dead. But for many of us widows, we don't believe it ourselves. I knew Bob was looking out for me when I found his credit cards still in his wallet in his top dresser drawer, so that I could find the phone numbers for Discover and Visa to stop the use of my cards when they were stolen. A widow who was nervous about freeway driving and one particularly difficult exit, wrote that the day she spent the entire trip worrying about how she was going to get to the off-ramp, she found, when she got there, that there was no traffic at all, and off she went. It was her husband looking after her, she wrote.

An e-mail came on a Monday from another Phyllis who had been married to another Bob. Her sixty-fifth birthday was to be that week, and she decided to buy herself a gift — from Bob. He had always enjoyed giving her gifts, and she knew he would want her to have something special for this special birthday. She went to the mall, and, at the first store she went into, found a beautiful dress, a perfect fit, bought it, and knew he would have approved a purchase made after just one stop.

One woman found help for herself in a marvelously unique way: she decided to learn to play pool, and she became so proficient that she joined a pool-playing group that went to Las Vegas to compete for the national championship. That group of nineteen to eighty-year-olds all became such compatible friends that on New Year's Eve they shot pool from five p.m. until eight a.m.

I had a good laugh when I heard from a woman who, taking a page from my book, learned how to pay her own way when she was out to dinner with two couples who kept picking up her check. My advice had come from a woman I know who says, quietly, to the waiter, "I would like a Beefeater martini and my own check, please." Quite accurately, the e-mail writer had said to the waiter the night before, "I would like a Dewars on the rocks and my own check, please," yet somehow she received the bar bill for all five people. "Don't you love it?" she wrote.

Just today, the mailbox held three completely different letters, each a special treasure. I opened the thicker packet first, and it was a CD written and recorded by a devoted granddaughter, who captured the essence of her grandmother's widowhood by singing softly as she played the guitar, "She's a widow who stares at the TV, misses her mate . . . misses her date."

With the music quietly playing in the background, I opened the next letter and a picture fell out. This woman and her husband had not only known the Sid Gillmans some twenty years ago in La Costa, California, but had been to many social events with them. (In *It Must Have Been Moonglow*, I had told of reading a *New Yorker* book review that mentioned Sid Gillman. He was the coach of the San Diego Chargers, and my football hero at Ohio State when I was a teenager.) She had taken the trouble to find an old photo of this group of friends, had Kinko's zero in on Sid, and sent me the copy of his picture. "I got the same reaction reading your book at three a.m. that you got reading *The New Yorker*," she writes. One degree of separation.

The third letter did not even need to be read; the message of love was right there on the envelope. Printed along with the return address was a one-and-a-half-inch-square photo of a smiling couple, he in a World War II leather aviator jacket, and handwritten below, " 'The way we were,' October 1945." On the reverse side of the envelope my correspondent had printed, "What I miss is connubial bliss." (Of course, I read the letter itself, too. This is a seventy-nine-year-old woman with a charming sense of humor.)

Awake and alone, in the wee small hours of the morning, widows have written me six- and eight- and ten-page letters. They have included poems and prayers and newspaper clippings — obituaries and daughters' bridal photos — and *handkerchiefs*.

A columnist whom I read quite faithfully once wrote a story about a boy who thought he might pay his way through college if every reader of the column sent him a penny. Well, he received not only enough for four years' tuition but, with the excess, he made a nice charitable contribution somewhere.

I only just mentioned, in my *Moonglow* book, that handkerchiefs were obsolete — I could not find a store that sold them — and, immediately, those same caring, loving people out there began to send me handkerchiefs. I have twenty-some new handkerchiefs, the names of two stores where they are available for purchase, and proof that goodness and benevolence still exist today, even as we wage war against terrorists and pray for peace in the Mideast.

Six of the handkerchiefs were a gift at Christmastime from the dear, young wife of my only nephew. She is a veritable old-handkerchief connoisseur, collecting them at yard and garage sales and flea markets. These are (near) antique, and I am almost afraid to use them. But I do. For our family in-gathering on July 4, she brought me yet another wonderful handkerchief, with "Wede" (my grandmother name) embroidered on the corner. How lucky can I be?

I had another gift of three brand-new embroidered beauties from a young friend whose family still lives in Wales. Whenever she goes to visit, she buys a few gift boxes of lovely Irish linen handkerchiefs to bring home and have on hand for future gift giving. Trouble is, there are so few people who still use handkerchiefs; thus she had a box at the ready when she read *Moonglow*.

One other multiple gift I received was part of a marvelous memory. The house our children grew up in was on a leafy street in what we all believed was an idyllic community, if you were foolish enough not to look too deeply below the surface or beyond its boundaries. It was the world of Ward and June Cleaver and Dick-and-Jane first readers, where "safe and secure" was taken for granted. We left the back door unlocked so that Bill, the milkman, could come in, check the refrigerator, and leave what we needed — and his company would send the bill at the end of the month. He could be sure that I would pay the total submitted; I could be sure he would charge only for the butter and milk (and even orange juice, I think) that he left. Remember the fifties?

The children didn't even have to cross a street to find friends. They could cut through the backyards, and there was a neighborhood full of kids whose houses fronted on the next leafy street to the north of us. We moved from that house thirty years ago.

And then a package with two beautiful embroidered handkerchiefs arrived in the mail from Colorado, from a long-ago little girl who had lived on that street and who was now a widow, much too young, with two children of her own. I wrote to thank her, of course, and she called me — and we talked for an hour. We reminisced about her brothers and the Greene "children" and the other neighbors. As we talked, I could see a slim, wiry, active eight-year-old with long, blond hair, and she remembered that I had once called her mother to send her back to our house to help clean up the mess she had made in Tim's room. (Puzzle pieces all over, as I began to recall.) I was horrified to be reminded that I had done such a thing. It seems there must be something to this selective memory theory.

That accounts for twelve handkerchiefs. The others were from total strangers. Some were in the envelope with a letter without even mentioning the enclosed gift. Some told me whether they had bought it, or owned it, or had embroidered it. One, in a square envelope made by closing the flaps on four sides, was really a valentine. The kindness of strangers, indeed. I am humbled and gratified and teary as I write.

To do justice to the beauty of the correspondence, I ought to quote verbatim. (I only do so after requesting and receiving express permission on a few selected letters.) I consider this personal mail, communication between friends. Friends respect each other's privacy. And I am respectful beyond measure of each and every person who did me the honor of writing.

Reach Out, Try to Touch

Tonight, every single communications appliance in this house is broken. I was born much too soon and ill-equipped. I am trying to be of this world, but each time I change long-distance carriers, or cell-phone programs, or computer platforms or browsers or whatever they are called, I dig the hole deeper.

Two weeks ago, I had a moment of revelation about the numbers and size of the various bills I was paying. Some of them were just a line item on my credit card and escaped my attention. Some were being automatically deducted from my checking account and, of course, they didn't appear on my radar screen until the checkbook became completely unbalanced. Others, I just paid as the price of living in the twenty-first century. (The twenty-first century, egad!) Put them all together, they spell m-o-n-e-y, and I was sure I could be more creative in the way I reached out and touched. First off, I got rid of Herself, old Ma Reach-Out-and-Touch. Talking to an

AT&T computer in English, and asking it questions that it automatically answers, is annoying. How can it possibly anticipate (i.e., be programmed for) every question that anyone might pose? ("How many miles is it to the moon," I should have asked.) I am reluctantly willing to follow prompts for half an hour, but if I am going to have a Q&A, I want the "A" to be real and alive.

It is a stretch to say I am reluctantly willing to follow prompts, but there are times . . . Worse yet is to call, say, to order some flowers for an ailing friend and be greeted by the ever-cheery, "All of our operators are helping other customers," and then comes the music, interrupted by the hard-sell messages directly antithetical to what is happening to you at that moment. You hear how Posy Rosy can make any occasion special, how their carefully trained gift-care specialist can meet your every need, that the knowledgeable customer-care representative will be right with you, that they thank you for your patience and they invite you to join as a preferred member. Finally, a real, live, ill-informed, unresponsive, unwilling expert answers. Or in utter aggravation, you think you will use a famous FedEx florist delivery service, only to have their inventory unable to keep up with the orders, so that you (and I have) in desperation ordered ten different items only to find, as soon as you say "Okay," the patient operator sees on her screen "No longer available."

And where are these Talk America people who have been courting me every dinnertime, just as I pick up my fork? I have said, "No thank you," "No thank you" until I just said, "Not interested" and finally just, "No," and hung up. Yet, now I want to say "I am interested" or "Tell me more," and I cannot find them!

Well, how amazing. Talk America has morphed from (or is that into?) "Member LD" of America Online. In fact, they had an interim name change that I missed. But, aha!, I tracked them down and asked them to sign me up. They are competitive: if you spend at least five dollars in a month, it is 3.9 cents a minute, no monthly fee. This gives me 128.20512 minutes a month to call all over the country, but that will be hard to do because I changed my Cingular cell-phone calling plan, too.

I had been paying around $30 for 100 minutes a month, until I saw the full-page ads for 3,000 minutes of unlimited night and weekend calls, plus 150 anytime minutes, for $35, so that seemed a worthwhile extra expenditure. Because I believe in instant gratification, and because Cingular has a store next to my beauty parlor, I was right on site to urge them to revise my contract. That modest cost-enhanced plan should kick in any day now. So, for the next year, I'll call anybody anywhere. Just tell me your number. I have 3,250 cellphone minutes a month to chat with you, which translates into 39,000 minutes a year. You may need to get in line, though. That is only 2,600 fifteen-minute calls. And whoever spent only fifteen minutes trying to reach your computer service or your energy utilities or your airlines? (This week, there was a long article in the business section of our daily paper, decrying/ explaining this very problem. The American Customer Satisfaction Index that had been compiled by the University of Michigan Business School has verified that the automobile industry rates the highest and the airline industry the lowest in waiting-time satisfaction. Doubtless, the responses depended directly on whether the person surveyed had just tried to call to make an appointment to have their tires rotated or to make an airline reservation.)

With all the fabulous features available

on my Nokia cell phone, I have only mastered the ability to call out. I do not know how to receive a call. I have had many an impatient teacher tell me to push this button, then that, then this again, and . . . there you go. Their hands are quicker than my eye, and their techno-knowledge is too internalized.

One day, in California, at lunch with my granddaughter, I learned that I should always have my cell-phone keys in a locked position. Locked? How? Why? Well, it appears that a husband hugging his wife as he comes home in the evening can activate the speed dial on the phone in his pocket, and the person who has been inadvertently dialed then hears the ensuing conversation between husband and wife. It struck me as a very unlikely scenario, until that very afternoon: I was back at the hotel resting and my dial-locked phone rang, and where would a grandmother look for an "unlock button"? I knew the call had to be from my granddaughter, because no one else — no one — knows my cell-phone number. Shortly, she called on the room phone. She was at the beauty parlor and had sat on her cell phone, on my newly installed speed-dial number, on her unlocked keypad! Beware!

The next morning, I was sitting in the sun and called a California friend with whom I really wanted to visit. Her husband told me she was busy at that moment but would call me back in five minutes. I gave him the cell-phone number. I was still mightily confused about the receive mode for her incoming call. I asked every group of people at the pool how to set the phone. (I longed for any fifteen-year-old boy; they all know about these arcane matters.) When minutes later the phone actually rang, all the sunbathers applauded our combined triumph.

This "global" calling (within the continental United States) I had planned got off to an inauspicious start. AT&T left me before Talk America joined me; therefore, tonight, I am without any land-based long distance at all. It is Saturday and all business offices are closed until after the holiday. That would really be all right, I guess, because I have my new copier and fax machine to send New Year's messages far and wide — except for the fact that the fax screen continues to display "paper jammed."

Fast forward to post-weekend heavy traffic on Hamilton Road as I drive to return the machine. Of course, I cannot fit it into the precisely molded Styrofoam packing that kept all the many parts of the machine in precisely the right small spaces. Box and machine sit separately on the backseat of the car as I plan which one I can carry into the store and which one I can ask a clerk to go retrieve. I carry the box — because the universal code is some proof that I bought it at this store — and the clerk incredulously asks me if I want her to reach into my car . . . without me at her side. As I explain that getting from the car to the store, and then back to the car and to the store again, is what I cannot do, she reluctantly goes to get the fax/copier. A technician examines it. "The paper jams," he says. "I think it is defective." I buy another (more expensive) model and head for home.

Now it is time for the cable guy to install a new cable so I can have a high-speed connection for my computer, thus allowing me to be online and not tie up the phone line. Two guys later — and a much more complicated route into the house for the additional cable line, including drilling a new outlet in a closet where I would rather not have it — I wait for the technician who need only connect the modem to the machine. How reassuring to hear that the entire high-speed system is temporarily down; and, since they and I cannot find a time convenient for both of us for the next day (which is a Friday), someone will arrive between nine and one on Monday.

Just for the record: before I had evaluated my needs to fax and copy (I literally have none), I had thought it imperative that I own a fax/copier/telephone-answering machine with caller ID. Add to this record that I returned it — because it was impossible to program — and bought a plain old telephone with answering machine. I set and reset the clock, but a gremlin automatically changes "a.m." to "p.m." while I sleep, so when I retrieve my messages you cannot believe who calls me at three a.m! I swear my rabbi's secretary wouldn't do that!

My local carrier phoned me four days in a row — four days! — to urge me to buy "private messaging," which helps a subscriber get around blocked calls, and when I foiled them on that little merchandising ploy, they called the next two days to urge me to use their "local" long distance. Please leave me alone!

With a panoply of devices fit for a multinational company, and an aversion to the whole cell-phone/bottled-water culture that surrounds me like shrink-wrap, I say into the aerosphere, "Hello operator. Are you there? Are you there?"

My Life at Bear Creek Orchard

Lord, thou knowest that I am growing older. Keep me from becoming talkative and possessed with the idea that I must express myself on every subject. Release me from the craving to straighten out everyone's affairs. Keep my mind free from the recital of endless detail.

Give me wings to get to the point. Seal my lips when I am inclined to tell of my aches and pains. They are increasing with the years and my love to speak of them grows sweeter as time goes by.

Teach me the glorious lesson that occasionally I may be wrong. Make me thoughtful but not nosy — helpful but not bossy.

With my vast store of wisdom and experience it does seem a pity not to use it all. But thou knowest, Lord, that I want a few friends at the end.

(A VERY SAVVY) ANONYMOUS AUTHOR

It was summer of 1943 that the newly activated 91st Infantry Division went on maneuvers for two months in the area around Bend, Oregon, some four hours away from Camp White. Medford became a town of lonely women, mostly new brides like me, with not much to do. A highlight of the afternoon was to walk "downtown" to Roxy Ann's and have a piece of the best apple pie à la mode I have ever eaten. Filling but unfulfilling. I needed a job and I applied to the largest employer around, home of Harry and David's Bear Creek Orchard, the original Fruit-of-the-Month.

They needed pear packers.

I was short on dexterity but long on availability and, in what I optimistically considered a signing bonus (long before signing bonuses were a fact of life), we were to work outside in the magnificent Oregon sunshine. I keep trying to reconstruct in my mind the exact configuration of the revolving boxes. I remember I stood in the middle, more blind mouse than cheese standing alone. The famous Royal Riviera Pears were in a bin to my right, the wrapping papers in front of me, and the wooden boxes with Harry and David's pictures on the blue labels were circling around and around on a conveyor belt outside of my station (I think). The object was to pick up a pear with your right hand, grab one of those flimsy little papers, wrap it around the pear, and lay it gently in the box with the logo (then called, in plain language, a label) as the box passed by. Theoretically, you would have another pear ready as the next box arrived, and you then laid this pear down so its stem end was next to the fruity end of the one already nestled. It wasn't easy! I lasted three days.

Management (Harry? David?) then decided they could use me in the "Hold" system. That summer, I *was*, in fact, the "Hold" system. *In toto.* As orders for future deliveries came in, I made notes, by hand, of the customer and all pertinent information on a 3x5 file card. Sometimes I had to go downstairs and cross-check what I had in the black-mottled cardboard file box with information in a set of real metal filing cabinets. My file was arranged by months; and, I assume, when I left at the end of my short stint, someone used that information to send "Pearsnapples" to the proper recipient on the proper date. I will never know.

I hope Harry and David (the company) kept a soft spot in its corporate heart for me; I certainly have one for it. Each holiday season, I look at the seven hundred catalogs that arrive with beautiful food gift ideas and, invariably, I order something from Fruit-of-the-Month. They make it easy by enclosing my list from the year before, so all I need do is give them the proper item number — they have the names and addresses — and then I give them the charge card number, and we are done. Or we are supposed to be done. Or the poor operator believes she is done. Each year, I promise myself that I will say "Thank you," and hang up. And then it comes pouring out of my mouth and, out of that soft spot in my heart, I begin and I cannot stop myself.

"Can you believe that sixty years ago, I was your original hold file?" "Does it seem possible that file card and pen have grown to computers and networks and platforms, nationwide delivery centers and databases and . . . ?" "Oh," she will say. "Oh." Encouragement enough for me. I explain how we lived on Ivy Street, in a white-frame, single-story house that had been converted to apartments. (Not apartments, exactly, I tell her. More like a divided-up first floor with three front doors.) Norma and Stan lived next door with Keith and Thyra. After the war, Keith went on to become a senator from Nebraska — or maybe, I clarify, maybe it was Montana — and once when we had been in Florida, we drove home through D.C. and had dinner with them in a dining room open only to members of Congress and their guests; and there was a terrible snowstorm and we were almost stuck, but we had to get back to our children; and we drove home through snow four feet deep. I stop for breath and operator #00 thinks she is almost free, but I have yet to tell her how Thyra and Keith and Norma and Stan took turns with having a real bed — one week in the bedroom, one week on the couch in the living room. And, I say, "Guess what? Thyra came over to use our phone so Norma wouldn't hear her conversations." "Really," says operator #00. "Really?"

I have asked before about the library that was up at the corner, about the Medford Hotel. I know Camp White, that old camp in the Agate Desert, is gone, that the old 91st is no more, that my Medford and hers are two entirely different places. Do I keep talking and talking to bring my beautiful experiences alive for her, or to keep that memory bright for me? How many impatient shoppers, waiting for the next available operator as I ramble and ramble, have hung up and called Wolferman's and chosen #3054, the delectable scone sampler basket, as a gift, instead? I would hope that to my old Bear Creek friends, shedding years by sharing memories is worth a few lost pear sales. Isn't it?

Pavlov, Gwen Ifill, and Me

Washington Week has been a favorite program of mine for years. I began watching early on, was always impressed by Paul Duke's diplomatic style controlling the correspondents, thought Ken Bode was a fine and worthy replacement, and am thrilled that Gwen Ifill — a woman with know-how, credentials, and charm — became the moderator in 1999. *Washington Week*, the longest-running public-affairs program on the air, is in very good hands.

Rate the correspondents good, better, best — as you will. The news, in and of itself, is compelling and scary enough to keep us on the edge of our seats. My problem is that I don't watch from a seat: Friday night, the end of the somehow always-busy week, is when I get into bed and eagerly turn to PBS at eight o'clock. My electric blanket has been turned to low as I take my early shower; I have propped my pillows and have turned on the bedside light. I settle down; I hear "Good evening, this is *Washington Week* and I am . . ."; my eyes close, my head drops, and I sleep the most beautiful, comforting, dreamless sleep in the world — Friday after Friday after Friday. I'm sure Gwen doesn't mind; I mind. She probably would not begrudge me those minutes of heavenly rest, with the light on and the TV blaring, those minutes that escape me so often during the night. But I really want to hear the program. Even knowing what I am missing, I cannot help myself. It is a conditioned reflex born of many weary Friday nights, and I am like one of Pavlov's dogs. I truly would like to change this pattern, but I have come to treasure that sleep, which is a rare commodity.

We all have our ingrained habits that have become part of who we are. When I am on a plane and they come around with the beverage cart, I order Mr & Mrs T, without the vodka. I never ordered a Bloody Mary on a plane, so that doesn't explain it. I don't keep the mix in the refrigerator at home. It is just what I do midair. When I nap in the afternoon (and I do, I do), I lie on my back on the couch in the living room and my mind knows it's time to grab those few winks. My nightly sleeping is always on my right side; the right side of my hair is always bedraggled, but that is my only fetal position-of-choice — or, rather, of habit.

I once knew a man who had a consistent, unvarying shaving pattern. He shaved something like Monday morning, Tuesday night, then Thursday morning, etc. No matter his business or social schedule, he would not deviate from this shaving plan. He was either appropriately clean-shaven or crudely bewhiskered. How he appeared at a conference or a party or his childrens' graduation was the luck of the razor's edge. I was a young woman when I heard this probably apocryphal story, and I was told it either to teach me the value of sticking to my game plan, the foolishness of being stubborn or, more likely, to help me accept that an ingrained habit can become a conditioned reflex. Take your pick: this man was a Pavlov dog. We program ourselves.

Nora Ephron, Wellesley '62, the talented journalist, writer (*Heartburn*), and director (*When Harry Met Sally*), was invited to deliver the commencement address in 1996. Her remarks were pithy, to the point, and humorous; she assured the graduates that they could "have it all," but not all at the same time. As I read the address in the alumna magazine, the words that jumped out at me were about a game she played while waiting for a table in a restaurant (that's her life) and which I have been doing ever since, while waiting in line for the grocery checkout (that's my life). She thinks of five adjectives to best describe herself to herself. As a college graduate, she would have written, "ambitious, college graduate, daughter, Democrat, single." Ten years later, the adjectives had all changed: "journalist, feminist, divorced, New Yorker, funny." In 1996, they had changed once again, to "writer, director, mother, sister, happy." Play the game sometime. Try to be honest with yourself. I know I was a student, bride, army wife, mother, community volunteer, grandmother, widow and, now, author. It is the "ambitious," "funny," "happy" adjectives that take more thought, because we need to recognize that those words can mutate as often as our occupation. We do not see ourselves as others see us, so that would be a good game, too: compare your list with a longtime friend; they are not going to be the same. We are in control of most of those defining adjectives. What power!

What we choose to do on a daily basis can become rote. If our days have been defined by a Pavlov-without or a Pavlov-within, we, and all of those who know us, will find us very predictable. The secret to shedding years lies in our ability to change those predispositions if that change is an improvement.

Dear Gwen: this week I am going to watch *Washington Week* in a (not-too-comfortable) chair.

Post It

Choose any dividing line, no matter how arbitrary, and people can always be found on one side or the other: women who use lipliner and those who don't; people who include anchovies as part of their "with the works" pizza and those who don't; those who sleep naked and those who don't; and (I actually knew a family who allowed this) kids who take Coca-Cola to school in their lunch-box thermoses and the rest of the kids who don't (and "got milk"). And then there are folks who have bulletin boards and — well, I just can't imagine it, but there are — people who don't!

We all, perhaps unwittingly, define ourselves by those things we choose to keep. Keeping them says we care about them. Caring about them says who we are. We hear so often that just to look at the books on the shelves in a stranger's library will outline the profile of that person. Fiction writers often use descriptive lists to define the nature of their characters, because in a good list you can paint in many dimensions. If you have read *Franny and Zooey*, I am sure you have not forgotten Mother Glass opening the mirror-faced door of the Glass-family medicine chest. The words that followed had the flow of poetry. "Before her," J. D. Salinger wrote, "in overly luxuriant rows, was a host, so to speak, of golden pharmaceuticals, plus a few technically less indigenous whatnots." He goes on, then, to name every item in the cabinet, from iodine and Mercurochrome to Sal Hepatica and two Gillette razors, one Schick injector razor, a small unlabeled box of glycerine suppositories . . . "two seashells . . . the strapless chassis of a girl's or woman's gold wristwatch . . . a girl's boarding-school class ring with a chipped onyx stone . . ." There is a good deal more, but even from this sampling, you begin to know the Glass family.

When Julian asks, in Erica Jong's *Any Woman's Blues*, what people eat, what they should have in their refrigerator, Leila tells him: "Raisin bran, milk, bananas, coffee, apples, sliced turkey, rye bread, mayonnaise, mustard, a barbequed chicken, tuna fish, butter cookies, chocolate ice cream, aspirin, Valium, yogurt." Now we understand something about Leila.

Deasey, the drunken boss of Kavalier

and Clay, whose *Amazing Adventures* are told by Michael Chabon, is best described by the contents of his desk, moved from the old Kramler Building to the new respectability of Rockefeller Center. The desk drawers "are stocked with fresh ribbons, blue pencils, pints of rye, black twists of Virginia shag, clean sheets of foolscap, aspirin, Sen-Sen and Sal Hepatica. . . . This — these fifty square feet of new carpet, blank paper and inky black ribbons — was the mark and clear summation of what he had attained."

If my psyche were the object of an archaeological dig, my bulletin board would yield the clues with which to begin. The items found there, and the strata in which they can be found, reveal, like the rings on a tree trunk, both my age and my history. Some of them have been there since the beginning of time; they are the foundation. There are a second and third layer, and the brand-new, most-recent additions are on top, often for the briefest of stays. Let me describe, now, what I have thumbtacked there, if you can bear to know me any better than you already do.

The oldest item, by far, is two life sketches, pencil drawings by our wonderful baby-sitter, Rosanna Penn, then in high school, most recently the illustrator who did the title page of *It Must Have Been Moonglow*. It shows our son Bob, age four, in feet-y pajamas, looking at his stash of 78 rpm plastic records; and, in the other panel, two-year-old Debby, almost hidden by the toy box she is trying to look into. This has been on so many bulletin boards through the years that you cannot even count the thumbtack holes along the sides.

Also, on that foundation layer are two extremely yellowed clippings. Not that I bothered to put a date on anything: the more yellowed gets the nod as the older of the two. (We will discount the quality of the paper on which each one was printed. It really doesn't matter the date, either. I kept them because they seemed timeless on the day I put them up; they still seem that way today.)

The first one is an Ellen Goodman column called "Must Women Operate the Family Switchboard?" She questions whether they must, but acknowledges that they do. The friend about whom she is talking "delivers peace messages from one child to another; softens ultimatums from father to son; explains the daughter to her father." The column talks about the Katharine Hepburn role in *On Golden Pond*.

51

"She placed herself between the angry, acerbic, viciously amusing husband — Henry Fonda — and the world. She was his buffer and his interpreter — to gas station attendants, the postman, their daughter."

Almost as yellow is this clipping from (it says) Mel's journal. It speaks so honestly to our always wanting to do our best and the obstacles we face. I think it is worth repeating in full.

Do everything right, all the time, and the child will prosper. It's as simple as that, except for fate, luck, heredity, chance, the astrological sign under which the child was born, his order of birth, his first encounter with evil, the girl who jilts him in spite of his excellent qualities, the war that is being fought when he is a young man, the drugs he may try once or too many times, the friends he makes, how he scores on tests, how well he endures kidding about his shortcomings, how ambitious he becomes, how far he falls behind, circumstantial evidence, ironic perspective, danger when it is least expected, difficulty in triumphing over circumstance, people with hidden agendas, and animals with rabies.

The final typed item is my school prayer, which I first learned in 1929. Adapted from an Episcopal book of prayers, it speaks to me today just as it did when I first enrolled at the Columbus School for Girls.

Watch over our school, O Lord, as its years increase, and bless and guide her children, wherever they may be. Let their hearts be warm with the flame of their youth's ideals, their faith unshaken and their principles immovable. Be thou by their side when the dark hour shall come to them; strengthen them when they stand, comfort and help them when they are weak-hearted, raise them up if they fall; and grant that all may grow in grace, and departing from ungodliness, may serve thee in pureness of living and truth.

Now we begin our upward climb. Stratum two is, primarily, columns by our son, Bob, and our daughter, DG Fulford. They speak about Ted Williams, a member of the honorary team voted to be the best ball players of the century; in a column headlined "The Tissue-Thin Decisions That Define Who We Are," the decision to just get by or do our best; and Bob and my busy life in Florida, when the dance we all do throughout our life turns out to be almost the best dance — the senior prom. One tells about my appearance on the *Today* show, and Katie Couric's kind call to my son. One is by Tracy Kidder, part of a review of a book (my little snippet of the clipping has excised the book title, but I wanted to keep the thought): "It's a little more elegant than Kant, actually. He says what's right is right and what's wrong is wrong, and the state of your internal being doesn't matter. You do the right thing even if it makes you feel bad. The purpose of life is not to be happy but to be worthy of happiness." I know exactly when I put it there, which child it was meant to encourage.

Next up is a sheet of Christmas stationery I had printed at Kinko's, with pictures in the upper-right and lower-left corners. In both, the three children and I are dressed in our best. The 1958 photograph was to run with a newspaper story about my heading the residential division of United Way. I hardly recognize myself with my dark hair and my smooth skin, but those well-behaved children are unmistakably Bob and Debby and Tim. The other picture was done by a professional photographer who, as a surprise, had been sent by my dear and loving nieces to a restaurant where the four of us were having a celebratory dinner for my eightieth birthday. Each of us was faking having a good time for the sake of each of the others. My husband was too much absent from that table.

I used the other three pieces of the stationery to write a note to each of my children's families with a Christmas check. I had not had the heart to go shopping. What a lot of history could have been written in that space between the two pictures. What a lot of history was written between the lines of my few words of love and season's greetings.

This is the same layer where the cartoons sit. My not-too-kind favorite is of a man standing behind his office desk, looking at an appointment book, and saying on the phone, "No, Thursday's out. How about never — is never good for you?" And the other is of two middle-aged women walking out the door of what might be a resort hotel, one saying to the other as they pass two old people sitting on a settee on the porch, "They don't have the secrets to anything — they're just old."

Now currently on top are reminders of

my visit to Steamboat Springs, Colorado. I have the *Steamboat Pilot* newspaper picture of my granddaughter Hannah's sixth-grade English class gathered all around me after I had visited them and talked to them about writing and publishing. There is also a downloaded picture from my son, Tim, of grandson Tucker facing off against captain Cammi Granato of the United States women's hockey team who, on their way to Salt Lake City, played an exhibition game with the Steamboat Braves.

As I was sitting down to my Uncle Ben's rice bowl last evening, I could see through the door to the deck that the forsythia are beginning to bloom and that my yellow finches are back at their feeder, eating the Nigerian thistle I had just put out for them.

There probably is an ethereal, illusory connection between the yellowed clippings and the yellow finches, but I will just accept the reality that they are all part of this long life I am privileged to enjoy.

There Will Never, Ever Be . . .

Another you. Of course, we all know that old truism, "Never say never," but for many of us widowed very late in life, it seems safe to say "never." I am happy for lonely people who, having lost a husband or a wife, find a new life and a new mate, renewal and contentment. For me, though, I think, Act I was the entire play, an act impossible to follow.

At a certain juncture, we grow comfortable in our widowhood. We would not have chosen it, but we find ourselves accepting that that is who we are.

I was at a lovely dinner party one night, a farewell for a friend who was moving out of town to a retirement community near her daughter. There were twenty-some people there; twenty widows and four men, excluding the host and his grown children. I was chatting with my dinner companion, a woman widowed young. Just that day, she had been on the telephone with another woman, whose husband had died two weeks before, who recounted that she had been out to dinner with two couples and had been screaming inside through the entire evening.

In the beginning, it truly is agonizing. I then told my dinner companion the story of my first night out after Bob died. Four of us, widows all, went to a movie and dinner. As I sat in the restaurant, with good, good friends, lifetime companions, I felt the most overwhelming sense of despair. Is this it? For the rest of my life? I was despondent and forlorn — screaming inside.

Yet, here I was discussing that deep emotion at a dinner party, as if it had happened to someone else. Had I been healed by that remedy called "compound tincture of time" (a phrase our pediatrician used years ago)? Am I resigned to being widowed? I think I am, and with resignation comes a certain peace and the strength of knowing that, for the time being, I can count on myself. It is a lifesaving revelation.

This is a solution for me. There is, of course, the flip side: the happiness that others find in reconnecting, in starting over with a new and loving mate. Quite a number of letter writers, responding to *Moonglow*, were remarried widows, extremely happy. Love, as Cahn and Van Heusen wrote, and so many of my correspondents agreed, "is lovelier the second time around . . . Just as wonderful with both feet on the ground." This was the message from women who had had both happy and unhappy first marriages; they were either rediscovering the joy of matrimony, or finding it for the first time. As we all grow older (and so often feel younger), a new relationship is life-affirming and often a tribute to the success of the first marriage. Yet whatever songs of love are playing, *Moonglow* is on the turntable of my mind. (I know about tapes and discs and DVDs; for me, the music still goes round and round on the turntable!)

Among my acquaintances, there is good news and bad news in the ever widening, interlocking circles of single women. From in town and afar, I hear happy talk — of a woman who plans to be married to a long-time friend with whom she and her husband never lost touch, and stories of true romance begun on the Internet: from a chat room, to a connection, then meetings, and, ultimately, marriage. And the not-so-good news of other women who long for another chance at married life, who are lost and lonesome and defenseless without a husband. There is no one out there for them.

We find ourselves on this journey alone. We have some small control of our destiny. Options abound, yet we cannot always have what we want; we have learned that early in life. All we can do is seek our own best solution. As the great philosopher Yogi Berra told us: "When you come to a fork in the road, take it."

Merchants of Discontent

A few words on the economy from a consumer: why, why do the manufacturers keep tampering with their products just for the pleasure of tampering? That is not the reason, they will say. We are tampering to create something flashier, different, more appealing, something that will lure you to the counter or the showroom or — of all places — the manicure table. They do not even call it tampering; they call it innovation. When the new, improved product is truly new — or improved — that's the better mousetrap we long for. (I'm not knocking those new electrostatic dust cloths or new Crayola colors or the incredible TiVo system that allows your TV to do everything but calculate your taxes. It's those other changes, just to change, that can drive a buyer crazy.)

Take hosiery. I first had the grown-up thrill of wearing silk stockings in 1933 — stockings instead of little white cuff-turned-down socks. What some may remember of that year is that Franklin Roosevelt closed the banks; what I remember is my first garter belt. Seven years later, nylons were first shown at the 1939 New York World's Fair and caused a sensation — but nylon had to be used for parachutes, belts, and other gear during World War II, and so, for the duration, we were back to silk hose with the seam down the back. (I was happy. I thought silk much more fetching than this less sheer, man-made material.) By 1945, despite some of us diehards, tough, durable nylon became a worldwide staple. Women loved them. As nylon became more sheer and more flexible, manufacturers invented panty hose, so retail stores could use their space for more colors and styles, since there was no longer a need for the corsets that had held up the old thigh-high stockings.

Doris Kearns Goodwin I am not, but there is a valid reason to devote this much space to history, even if it is the short history of hosiery. We can all pretty well agree that the newer items that came along had attributes that made them superior to the ones that came before and more attractive to the buying public. Today's changes, un-fortunately, are not the presentation of better products; they are simply merchandising ploys.

So why am I annoyed when I go to buy a

new pair of hose? It seems that the names of the colors *and* the design of the package *and* the identification of the sizes change from purchase to purchase. What if you have been wearing "traveltan" since the birth of your third child? What if the package always had looked the same and the code number was the same, and then, out of the blue, the package is updated and good old "traveltan" has taken its last trip? *What is the point?*

Not to beat this same horse to an untimely death, but consider nail polish. Occasionally, I get a professional manicure, and for a long, long, long time I have liked a color called (believe me) "Beige-Jing." It was a soft, dusty rose that didn't draw attention to your hands but helped you look well-groomed, and it was very popular with ladies of a certain age, of whom my beauty parlor serves many. Suddenly, "Beige-Jing" has vanished (and has not been replaced by "Pea-King," either). It has been replaced by "Queen of Denial." So maybe they change these products just to show how clever they are with words! Of course, it doesn't really matter at all; but, for those women who liked it, *what is the point?*

A more nefarious example may be that

we read that Prilosec is only minimally changed to become Nexium; the same small difference turns Claritin to Clarinex. Both versions remain on the market; the generic is delayed that much longer.

Finally, in the "leave well enough alone" category, are the corporate name changes. No one would ever accuse me of having a power portfolio. It is, in fact, pretty mundane, and I do not understand the siren call of day trading, of buying-selling-changing-buying-selling. I am not a broker's dream client. What I have, I have; what is out there can stay there. I stay constant, yet some names in my monthly brokerage reports look unfamiliar. A lot of that has to do with buyouts and spin-offs, I know, but it seems that name changes for merchandising reasons also play a role. Plain old Houston Power & Light is now Reliant Energy; LePercq Net 1, L.P. has become Lexington Corporate Properties Trust; TXU was once, I think, Texas Utilities. Bright red, as always, in the commercials at the Masters golf tournament, was the umbrella of the Travelers Insurance Company. Except, of course, the Travelers were under the corporate umbrella of Citigroup, which also sheltered Citibank and Salomon Smith Barney and Primerica and CitiFinancial! And final insult of the year: Philip Morris is now Altria Group, Inc. Can you even imagine that little bellboy yelling, "Call for Al-Tria, call for Al-Tria"? How many Als staying in that hotel would rush to the house phone, having understood only the first syllable of the page? Even though stockholders are not standing and cheering for the performances of Coca-Cola and IBM, at least they know who they are!

To stay young, I need to accept all of these changes gracefully; to go with the flow; be cool. We all need to go forward, not back; four on the floor, not reverse. It would be foolhardy to wish for fewer choices, to want only beige, white, and black hosiery or only red, pink, or colorless nail polish. It is not too far a leap for us to move from such minutiae to thinking about how democracies and dictatorships differ, how earthshakingly important it is to have the freedoms that allow not only us to choose, but the merchants of discontent to make choices as well. (Although I do wish they would ask my advice!) So I shall hang on for the ride, knowing where I have been, not always sure where I am going — just forward.

The More Things Change

In mid-February, the notice from the grass cutters arrived. They sent their 2002 price list, with a pick-and-choose form for this summer's services, and I signed up for another year of our April-to-October relationship. Shortly thereafter, the pool people wrote asking me to choose the date on which I wanted them to "open." It seemed as if they had just "closed," but I shut my eyes and my mind, got out my calendar, shot an arrow into the air — it fell on my calendar, I didn't care where (apologies, Henry W.), and we have a mutually agreeable date.

We are approaching the season of my discontent, the season when all the tasks Bob once could do (or even I could do) have become the province of others. I am grateful for their help, for the offer of my daughter's friends to do some of the heavy lifting while I, almost morosely, think about how everything has changed. Then, looking through Bob's meticulous pool file — when did we usually open? how much did it cost? — I came upon something I had written for the family in 1988 and had a much-needed laugh. Of course, of course, nothing has changed (except the price).

Now that April in Ohio has again arrived, I want to share the whole, old ludicrous chronicle.

Your mother writes:

This is a chronology of things that have happened to us this spring. I'm not sure why I feel I need to write them down, but it does seem important, maybe because we have come out on the other side of it all, not any better but, truly, not too much worse, except for the $$$ down the drain.

At the end of March, we came home from the coldest Florida season in years. We found that the roof, having been damaged in a February ice storm, had leaked through in a number of places, including onto the living room carpet and through our bathroom ceiling. This entailed negotiating with the insurance company and scheduling with Roy for the drywall work and finding Douglas who had made our short list of recommended painters.

Before either of them could even get here, I was driving east on Main Street when the Whitehall Sunoco half-ton

67

wrecker rear-ended me. I was fine but the Taurus wagon was a mess and had to be towed in. It was going to be two weeks before the car would be ready, but our insurance did pay for a rental car.

On Monday, April 25, the motor to the pool went out. Daddy worked most of that afternoon and Tuesday morning, trying to pump the prime, carrying water, putting the garden hose in the intake, going up and down the incline between the hose spigot, the pool equipment, and the skimmer. By Tuesday afternoon, he called for help. Mallory Pools arrived, suggesting we might need a new motor, and we debated what would be best: invest in the motor or move all of the equipment down behind the pool house so that water to the filter wouldn't always be running uphill! During the working and walking and talking, Dad fell to his knees and was helped to the house by the pool men. That night, his blood-pressure readings kept going higher than our Timex Healthchek monitor could record. Wednesday morning, he went over to see Dr. Shell. By noon, he was in Mount Carmel East Hospital.

An EKG, a CAT scan, a carotid artery reading, and innumerable blood tests proved (inconclusively) that he had had a transient ischemia attack and the Holter monitor showed a spiking of the heartbeat called a PVC.

(Masheter called that my car was ready to be picked up. When I went to return the rental and drive mine to the hospital, the battery was dead. Masheter lent me another car.)

Friday evening, Dad was released from the hospital with three heart pills a day added to the four prescriptions he already takes. Plus aspirin. Mallory came and put in the new pool motor.

By Saturday evening, I was tired — and dirty. The paint was still wet in our bathroom where Douglas had worked the three days Bob was in the hospital. I ran a tub in the guest bathroom. It ran cold. We could not get the pilot to stay lit on the hot-water tank. I called Tim's house and the baby-sitter answered. I called Mary and Mike, our good neighbors, who arrived with a flashlight and a wrench. Good try, but the heater was definitely broken. A twenty-four-hour emergency service never returned our call. Sunday, we heated water on the stove to wash our hands and faces.

Mike, our always-reliable plumber, had

to make two trips on Monday because the first heater he brought was the wrong size. As he was here putting in the right-sized heater, I ran the disposal and it began to make an awful sound; the bearings had gone. So Mike put in a new disposal, too. Becky, the wonderful cleaning lady who comes on Monday morning, discovered that the globe-shaped light fixture in the downstairs bathroom was half full of water. Mike could not find the leak. (No one has found it yet. It must have been from that half-bath I ran on Saturday evening.)

By Tuesday, I had a cold, chills, aches, nausea — and stayed in bed. Douglas kept walking through the bedroom to finish our bathroom. Dad continued to be unnaturally exhausted, a result of the TIA, we guess. Dr. Shell guesses not. He diagnoses a bladder infection and prescribes sulpha. In the middle of Friday night, Dad wakes up with chills, a completely swollen face, and hives.

The sleepy MD on weekend duty, answering our call, presumes that it is a reaction to the sulpha and tells us to go to the office's first-come, first-served Saturday care. We are there first, we are served first, and the doctor agrees that it is a sulpha reaction and puts Dad on Benadryl as an antidote. For the next week, Dad is asleep more hours than he is awake. When he is awake, he still has hives and he itches.

As we sit by the pool during the week, we watch the water level drop. Dad marks it with a pencil every evening and goes to bed very early. May is passing. The pool people get a frantic call from us. Find the leak! — and sure enough they do, underground between the filter and the outlet. Enough concrete is demolished in the search that our next service call is to Concrete, Inc. (or something like that).

Exactly one month has passed since Bob's TIA. He seems to be less exhausted; our annuals are planted and mulched. Dad's niece and her husband are coming through Columbus on their way to a college reunion, and I invite the Columbus family for dinner. It is a pleasant evening, but I have a funny pain in my side and a lump I can feel.

I have always thought of myself as indestructible.

Dr. Shell sees me on Friday afternoon and sends me, immediately, to a surgeon who says he will operate on Tuesday on what he is sure is a vertical, incarcerated hernia. Tuesday he does the hernia; Wednesday he sends me home; Friday, the motor to the compressor fan in the refrigerator stops. The refrigerator is warm and my incision still hurts.

Glenn, the only authorized Sub-Zero repairman in town, cannot come out but (shall we call him) Joe, another refrigeration specialist, does. He puts in a new motor, which cools the food and sounds as if a giant 727 is revving up in the kitchen.

I have gingerly taken the steps on Sunday and am lying on the patio when Daddy tells me the pool sweep has broken again.

On Monday, Glenn makes a service call and charges a consultation fee to say that the new refrigerator fan motor is a 6-watt instead of a 2-watt, that it runs counterclockwise when it should — what? — run clockwise. Joe comes back to make the job right.

We wait for the pool people all week, with Dad phoning them daily. By the end of Thursday, he decides to take the pool sweep motor out himself and he does, not without a few problems. He takes it to a machine shop, and they have it ready for pickup on Friday afternoon.

As I write this, it is mid-June. The re-wired pool sweep motor has been installed. Everything seems to be in working order. The sky is blue and bright; the garden is beginning to bloom; I feel okay; Dad feels okay; we have cold food and hot water. How differently this all could have ended. We are terribly lucky.

"Sumer is icumen in/Llude sing cuccu."

In retrospect, this story has all the ingredients for a very silly sitcom. If I hadn't written it down, I would have forgotten so much of it. As I reread what I first recorded, it makes me smile. I'm not sure I was smiling a lot when we lived through it, but does it sound nutty to say that, today, it has become a good memory?

The Jingles and the Meanies

In the mid-nineteen-twenties, my mother and twelve other young matrons decided to organize themselves into a "formalized" group (membership was by invitation; I never knew who the choosers were — I just knew the chosen). They called themselves the Jingles, which was an abbreviation of jingle bell(e)s, and met at each others' homes for lunch and cards every Friday. The luncheons were not simple; the planning, at least in our house, was serious. These women were compatible but probably competitive, and by the time they had been meeting for ten years, they were, I thought, old. Their younger sisters formed their own group when they were young-marrieds and called themselves the Meanies, an abbreviation of meanie-cats. I suspected that such groups were to be found in cities everywhere. Water seeks its own level socially and, sadly, there are pecking orders and rules of the (social) game. The cycles of life change, but somehow the rules don't, big city or small town. Twenty years ago we read . . .

And Ladies of the Club; today *Divine Secrets of the Ya-Ya Sisterhood* is a runaway hit and a movie. Selectivity, cliquishness, and exclusivity sells.

This arbitrary judgment made by a group of people about their similarities seems, today, when we finally understand the importance of diversity, somewhat elitist. Yet it made for happy days between World War I and the Depression, and if no one else will identify my parents and their friends as a "great generation," I will do so now. Ten short years between World War I and the Depression — 1918 to 1929 — only a decade to cement friendships and embark on life's journey. They did their job well.

All of my mother's friends, the Jingles, are gone; there is one Meanie still living, age ninety-eight, in a retirement community but still driving and thriving and very much interested in the whole, wide world.

My own group, spontaneously begun around 1950, was oriented more to night than to day. (Our ladies' luncheons were at Howard Johnson's, if we could find someone to sit with the children while they napped.) We began to meet shortly after the men had come home from every theater of combat, representing all the services — brand-new civilians with the war behind us. With minimum originality, we named ourselves The Saturday Night Crowd. Not every Saturday, but for a long, long run, seven couples of us met at each others' homes after dinner for a few drinks, some talk, and a lot of laughter. Sometime before midnight, we ate and went happily home. We were Saturday Night Live before there was a *Saturday Night Live*. Of the original fourteen, four remain.

My daughter is finding her own group. With respect for the past, she calls these friends Mingles, related by blood or birth or the subjective unconscious, a Jungian memory of times known only third-hand. It is interesting to see.

The making of a friendship is an art. To discover a group of individuals that develops into a group of friends is a lost art. We tend to make our similar interests and concerns the focus, not our innate personalities. Thus we have soccer moms, brokers going out for a drink after work, and neighbors whose only connection is their lawn care. Nomadic as we have become, this is probably a good thing. At long last, we are moving past tribal cultures and ancient customs, moving slowly to understand the value of diversity.

Last week, I saw *The Women* on TV. It is

the Clare Boothe Luce play, written in 1936 and then produced in 1939 as a movie. It was a televised version of the 2001 Roundabout Theatre revival that I saw, and it is terribly dated and foolish, exaggerated in the acting and the posturing and, I hope, even the theme. To watch a group of über-rich women with nothing to do but shop, have affairs, and order the maids and nannies around, with gossip their aerobics, works as satire; as theater, I found it utterly boring. Contrast it with *The Bonfire of the Vanities*, whose characters are equally self-involved and contemptible. I wonder if the movie version will look old-fashioned and petty in 2060? The book, like the works of Jane Austen, will remain a comedy of manners for a long, long time, I think.

As our children and their children scatter across the country, they will develop their own groups born of like interests or vocations, less and less likely to have any connection to their history. There will be no luncheons: the mothers will all be working. Coffee and sweet rolls at midnight — how quaint. But in a quiet moment, I like to think of that gentle time of the Jingles and the Meanies, and thus I dedicate this chapter to Dorothy Marcus, the last Meanie standing. Cheers!

It Is Better to Give . . .

Around the middle of October, when the stores put up Christmas decorations, the flutter of anxiety in the pit of my stomach reminds me that I need to start making my holiday gift-giving lists. Not only have I kept (i.e., made) Christmas lists since the beginning of time, I have kept (i.e., not destroyed) them. I have filed the really old ones; only 1985–2001 are in the current notebook. I wonder, as I turn to the next blank page, if it isn't *better* to receive than to give. It may, indeed, be more *blessed* to give, as the Bible tells us, but take a small survey of mothers and grandmothers on the hunt at holiday time, list in hand. At six a.m., outside a crowded Kmart, amid pushing and shoving peers, for the privilege of purchasing one of the few Cabbage Patch Kids inside, you'll find, I think, that better/receive beats blessed/give.

Every year there is a single "hot" holiday item. I have probably been in the hunt for thirty-five of the last fifty, and each year it gets harder. The item is more scarce and the hunter is more weary, yet the hunter's heart is filled with even more love, and more recipients with more requests, as December follows December. We began with Bobby, Debby, Tim. They then begat Maggie and Amanda and Nick and Tucker and Hannah, and now we have added Chris and Caroline and Carter. At least, some of them are at an age that a small check is very acceptable. Yet, what is unbearable is the thought of a sad or disappointed child or grandchild, when the remedy for happiness is right there behind the wheel of the car: get in that car and go to *one more store.*

Once upon a time, there were safe Playskool toys, no television commercials, and preschool-size children not old enough to say "I need" or "Here's Santa's list." But, they all learn. They learn.

One year, in the mid-nineteen-fifties, every girl-child in Central Ohio yearned for a Little Red Spinning Wheel. By mid-November, there were none to be had. For love or money. Anywhere. The spinning wheel may have spun out pot holders or it may just have spun loops of cotton into a long braid; for my little girl and my brother's three little girls, it spun pure gold. Dreams of Rumpelstiltskin's wheel,

Rapunzel's hair. No stone was left unturned, no store unvisited, but the spinning wheel was gone . . . gone . . . gone. It so happened that my brother was in northern Ohio on business, and was working with a furniture store there, when he spied, in a corner, a small toy department and . . . eight spinning wheels! He bought them all and brought them home to my basement. Four were earmarked for us, one set aside for a friend's child suffering the same spinning-wheel syndrome; three were surplus. Almost instantaneously (how do black-marketeers communicate so quickly?), I began to get whispered phone calls: "I hear you have a Little Red Spinning Wheel," these mysterious suburban mothers said. I no longer remember who the three lucky children were but, Honest Abe that I am, I do remember I collected only what my brother had paid! Being a Santa's Elf is one of the most rewarding jobs in the world.

Over the years, besides being an elf, I have been a detective, a sleuth, a gumshoe, a private eye. I have almost always found my prey: the drum major's hat (made by my mother's dressmaker); the Barbie of the year, or her house, or her car; the American Girl year 2000 outfit — sold out by

80

catalog, found at the new retail store just opened in Chicago; a copy of the out-of-print book *Hans Brinker: or, the Silver Skates*. (This last was my idea, because Tucker is an ice-hockey aficionado. At Amazon, the Half Price bookstore, and the Village Bookshop, *Hans* was either too pricey or unavailable. I went to the computer, to my "Books and Criticism" forum. This group of book lovers are to be found online, on AOL, in SeniorNet. We have been meeting/posting for more than five years, ostensibly about books. We do recommend, review, and critique, but we have also grown to know, enjoy, and truly like one another. We are cyberspace friends, turning to one another in times of joy and sorrow. We send messages when one of us is ill; we give thanks for returned better health. These friends are a fount of information and good advice. I asked if anyone had a good source for finding *Hans* and received a copy as a gift from a friend who, moving, was weeding out books.)

There is always the moral-and-ethical question to consider. Are the clothes requested by the preteen what the mother or grandmother thinks proper? The answer never is "yes." I have learned that the classic jeans and modest top don't cut it;

you might just as well send the too-tight, satiny-looking pants. Loafers? Saddle shoes? Heaven forbid! Pale blue, with three-inch soles and a Velcro-strap closing can warm a pre-teen heart even as her feet freeze in the Colorado snow.

(I was interested to hear, on *Talk of the Nation*, a learned and academic discussion on the proper ways to influence the clothing decisions being made by the female eleven-to-fourteen set. During the call-in part of the program, one mother was adamant that we should not give up our "power," a word she used to define our obligation to help children make the right choices. One father was equally exercised because his twelve-year-old daughter wore thong underwear. I was driving home from a meeting where the superintendent of Columbus public schools had given her "State of the Schools" annual address. She can be proud of the measurable gains that have been made in her first year on the job; the challenges to close achievement gaps, improve attendance, and improve financial accountability remain, not to mention undertaking a massive building program for a large, urban district where the newest school was built twenty-five years ago. What a juxtaposition: fourth graders in thong underwear to fourth graders who cannot read!)

One of my favorite stories is of a boy, about age six, who was beginning to question who was the wondrous giver of Christmas gifts. He was a clever young fellow and decided he would tell Santa Claus that he wanted a drum, but also tell his parents. That way, secure in the knowledge that his loving parents would, of course, give him what he had asked for, one new drum under the tree would mean that it was his gift from Mom and Dad — that they and Santa Claus were one and the same, that there was no Santa to bring him a drum. He told his secret plan to his sister and she, wiser still at age eight, "ratted" on him, as he lovingly tells it, and told her parents. Lo and behold, there under the Christmas tree on December 25 were two drums; if one was from Mom and Dad, the other had to be from S. Claus. The *New York Sun* had it exactly right in 1897: "Yes, Virginia . . ."

Am I too heavily involved here with the commercial aspects of Christmas? That is the complaint all the psychologists, sociologists, and right-minded thinkers make every year. We all decry the commercialism even as we respond to the siren call of the catalogs and the ads. We know not to over-load the credit card, but Christmas is not about knowing, it is about feeling.

Christmas is not even my holiday. Love is. Celebrated daily. No matter the year, no matter the child, it is to warm our own hearts that we make the effort, over and over — with joy. To make a dream come true, to create a memory, to sprinkle a little fairy dust, to build a sense of promises kept, and to preserve a sense of trust: don't you push your way into that Kmart and emerge with a Cabbage Patch Kid, triumphant? Of course. What are mothers and grandmothers for?

As Time Goes By

Poolside, on Longboat Key, Florida, I came smack up against my past.

It was wonderful beyond words. A camp friend I hadn't seen in seventy years (seventy years!) was on Longboat for the weekend, and a mutual friend gave us the treasured gift of a short reunion. Freda (Freddie, in 1932) is every bit as attractive as she was at Camp Forest Acres. Wilmington, Delaware, I figured when we first met, must be the sophistication capital of the world if it produced Freddie. In the Nancy Drew series, I had been reading about worldly girls just like her, with her beautiful, artfully cut dark hair and those kind of "laughing brown eyes." Not only did she have that great haircut, but the boy who lived next door to her in Wilmington wrote her almost every day, and enclosed an eyelash. (When I reminded her of that glamorous fact, she didn't remember his writing her at all, but she did remember his eyelashes!) We were such good friends over the course of three summers, but then we lost track.

And here we were, old women, perhaps, by some definition; young women by the luck of the draw. In a tone of voice I casually use to ask, "What did you do today," I kissed her hello and said, "So what have you been doing for the last seventy years?" In less than an hour (her weekend was jam-packed), we covered one hundred forty years — her seventy and mine — recounted a little good news about mutual friends, and mourned the loss of two men who had played major roles in our very early lives. Under a beneficent, sunny sky, it is possible to be transported through time and space.

In the spirit of believe-it-or-not, I beg you to believe what happened the morning after I wrote the above paragraph. It happened. At eight-thirty a.m., my phone rang, and a woman's voice asked for Phyllis Harmon, my maiden name. "This is she," says I. On the other end of the line was a girl/woman from Toronto, a bunkmate in that same Cabin Seven at Forest Acres! Last winter, in Florida, I had spoken on the phone to a woman, Marilyn, whom I did not know but who had attended a gathering of old Forest Acres campers. She had related this to Yvonne, who now was calling me. Yvonne knew nothing about *Moonglow* and probably had not even thought of me in the years since she left camp in 1935. She hadn't even remembered my first name until Marilyn told her that I, like the American buffalo, still roamed the earth. She remembered my friend, Lois, much more clearly. I could report that Lois and I are still friends, and I could tell Lois that her indelible impression was still floating in the air from Fryeburg, Maine, to Canada and back to Ohio, winning her the Most Memorable Camper award, 1932. Yvonne and I talked for half an hour and promised to keep in touch.

A few weeks after Yvonne's call, another Toronto bunkmate, Roslyn, called from Montreal. She and Yvonne have stayed in touch, and her memories of camp in 1932 are vivid and complete. I thought I had all the details stored away in that special brain cell labeled Forest Acres, but she recalled a little song in German that I had taught all the group — *"backen backen* . . . something . . . *Kuchen"* — a song I have no recollection at all of ever knowing. We talked and talked. These renewals and reunitings are gifts I could never have anticipated when I first began to write in the winter of 1999.

There are such magic moments and, I

suppose, the older you get the better the chance. On that same Florida trip — in fact, it happened at lunch the noon of the day Freddie stopped by to visit — fourteen women had gathered, invited for a single reason: we had all attended the same girls' school in Columbus, Ohio. Only one other woman was from my class of '37. There were two from the class of '35; the rest were from the years between then and now — years when I was long graduated and on to college and marriage and life. What a bond we share! What a treat to be part of a group that holds firm — again, through time and space — through the shared memories and values of an institution. Next week, six of our class will be in attendance at our sixty-fifth reunion, where we shall sing of "classes and school days." And remember.

Not that remembering is all that easy these days. Once again, I am indebted to my online book group for a fine idea: for your "to do" lists, keep a stenographer's pad rather than small scraps of paper or small memo pads. (I have always been fond of those snitched from high-end hotel rooms; they are well-designed and lend a certain panache to a well-worn telephone table.) As you accomplish items on your list, cross them out but don't tear out the page. Flip it. Better still, date it and you will have a personal history.

Almost everyone has a particular calendar to which they are accustomed. Mine has been sold by one of the TWIGs of Children's Hospital for years; the plumed quill pen on the cover and the title "Social Capers" is identical year to year, and a clue to the etiquette of its genesis. Only the printing color varies. Spiral bound, 9" wide, 6" long, it shows one week to each page, each day divided into morning, afternoon, and evening. In a basement storage drawer, I have them neatly arranged, back to front, 1953–2001. Every meeting, every party, every dentist appointment is there. Every wedding, every funeral. In our family, where preserving family history is a business, this is a gold mine. Your collection of steno pads could be yours.

Mary, my next-door neighbor, is the youngest of four grown children. Her parents, a Lutheran minister and his wife, lived, after his retirement, in a house in another part of the state where lawn size demanded that it be cut by a riding mower. They rode the mower until they were both ninety-five. He also drove his car to come visit his daughter until that trip was as dangerous as the mower. At which point, they moved to a retirement community to be near Mary, always side by side. Last year, Mary's mother died. Now, Mary is reading her mother's diaries to her dad. Seventy years of diaries. She is learning about her parents' daily life — things she had never known: that they once played golf; about the measles and diseases of her older siblings; of her parents' circle of friends. A place where her father can re-visit so much happiness and where she can unearth the untold wealth of memories to pass on to her children.

More than forty years ago, long after Iris began her journaling, Harvey Schmidt and Tom Jones wrote what became the longest-running musical in the world, *The Fantasticks*. How many people can we figure have seen it? I never did, but the song "Try to Remember" often runs through my head. It can come to me out of the blue, or it can come as I deliberately think of it when I am having what has become such a cliche, a senior moment, when I "CRS (Can't Remember S____t)."

Try to remember and if you remember,
Then follow, follow, follow.

At the same time that we are following the memories to a different time and place, we hurry, hurry, hurry in this speeded-up world, so that as we ride to a meeting with a friend and listen as she gets three calls on her cell phone before we are even near our destination, we come home to four messages on our voice mail (two of them meaningless nuisances) and find, in a pile of unopened mail, an envelope on the back of which there is a message: *"EMERGENCY. Prepare for difficult times. Enroll in your Chase payment protector!"*

It is then, even as we thrive on the fullness of our lives, that we yearn for the years "when life was slow and oh so mellow," when we were schoolgirls or campers, when we looked at the world ahead as a long, tree-lined, beautiful road — a smooth, paved, easily navigated road. Today, as we look back, we know that we have traveled over busy freeways, amid cars that sped beside us and cut in front of us, almost beneath tractor-trailers that kept creeping up on us. We have taken a completely different journey — a completely different route — than the one on which we embarked. What a ride!

These Are a Few of
My Favorite . . .

Things: I was at the beauty parlor, reading *Lucky*, The Magazine About Shopping, a new, glossy monthly I had never seen before. There was a long article on how to clean out a closet so that what's left can be arranged in a neat, orderly fashion, and which included a list of five items you must own and seven rules on what makes an item disposable. Two hangers suddenly appeared dancing before my eyes, in front of the manicure table: on one, the yellow ball gown I wore to the first Symphony Ball, thirty-five years ago; and, on the other, the riding jacket from the 1933 horse show, where I fell off the horse and gamely got back on, in tears, but never attended the Frances Robbins riding academy again. (What a relief for my father, who might have been wishing that I would fall off the piano bench, too.) Magazine rules or not, the dress and jacket stay! As does the wool sweater with the farm scene knitted into the front — the blue clouds, the autumn trees, the peaceful, grazing sheep, the geometric fence, and the flowers down around the waist. Tim gave me the sweater at least twenty years ago; it has, of course, sentimental value, and it is still darn good-looking — even though there never seems to be a right time to wear it.

And I keep my bed jacket! It had been a birthday gift to my mother, and she didn't need it and passed it along. I loved it; I love it still. The fabric frog buttons have fallen apart, and it may or may not live through another washing — but, oh! the memories it carries. Most especially, I think of Wednesday nights when Bob went to his poker game and I read comfortably in bed, until he came home to report his losses. They always were losses. I think his pride was hurt more badly than his purse. Why is that a comforting memory? Like so many others, it just is.

One of the magazine rules is that you dispose of beloved items gradually to ease the pain of separation anxiety: you move them from the regular closet to a spare closet, and then, if you haven't thought about wearing them for a year, you move them to an even more remote spot, and then, if you still don't yearn for them, you can give them away! Well, the ball gown, no matter how hidden away — if it were practically unreachable (some people still have attics, I know) — can bring a smile to my lips. It stays. As my mother used to say, "It isn't eating anything."

Of course, we hang on to heirlooms, or what we mistakenly think are heirlooms. Just watch that long line of folks waiting to get in to the *Antiques Roadshow* program, carting what they think/hope/pray is valuable. Of course, the items we see on TV all *are* valuable. That's why they are on TV. How many people, do you think, go home disappointed, having found that the old pewter pitcher, supposedly brought west in a covered wagon with great-great grandmother was actually made in a factory in Taiwan in 1953?

I held on to our son Bob's little plastic 45 rpm records for a long time; but, of course, not long enough — two more generations, and they will have some value. Worse, I got rid of a very large, framed, original drawing of Superman — given to him by a wonderful Cleveland aunt and uncle of my husband's, it hung in Bob's bedroom for years; after he graduated from college and we moved to the house in which I now live, I just gave it to the Salvation Army or Goodwill or somebody! If my children feel that I disposed of part of their inheritance, just think how the children of the aunt and uncle feel. I won't even look at eBay to calculate the value.

Two other valueless/valuable things I own are nice, but not truly sentimental, not truly family memorabilia. Hanging in the back hall, near the garage door, is a wooden key rack, painted black, about twenty-two inches long, with six pegs on which to hang keys. It has moved from house to house with us; when the children were younger, they each had an assigned peg. Now I have it all to myself, yet I still manage to have a full key rack. Wherever I hang my hat (so to speak), so, too, will I hang that key rack. And I have a key ring on that rack that I have had since 1979, a sixtieth birthday gift from a friend. I am so used to the key ring that it is almost an extension of my hand. Clear plastic, more than three inches long, with my initials in bright blue, it is easy to find in my purse — and for parking lot attendants to identify me with my car.

Last week, I went into the lovely stationery store on Main Street that is owned by a woman who, early on, decided to start a small business in her home, and grew it into two thriving, upscale, gift-and-stationery stores. I had my key ring in my hand. "Oh," she said, "that is one of the first items I ever sold. I was selling mostly stationery, but I saw that at a gift show, and it was an instant smash." As she remembered, it was manufactured by a sign maker in Toledo, and it sold like hotcakes. I am not the only customer still using it. There I was, hurrying in to buy a birthday card, with my keys in my hand, and as she saw it, a deluge of memories flooded through both of us. In that few minutes — seconds — we each recalled who had bought it from her, given it to me, how she started her business, what journeys I have embarked upon with those keys. Much of your life can flash before your eyes with very little provocation. And so I ask: can a plastic key ring become an heirloom? It seems that it can.

Along with the ball gown and the riding jacket and the sweater, my heirs are going to have to figure out how to divvy up all of the above.

Divvying up: it is a process that has caused family problems for generations. Even if siblings have lived in love and harmony for years, the hurt of breaking up the home of a parent often leads to more hurtfulness. There are often-repeated stories about arguments over the grand piano or the diamond brooch or, as in Eudora Welty's *The Optimist's Daughter*, the breadboard. I have not given this a lot of thought, because my brother's family and mine did it so easily and lovingly when my mother died. Cousins compromised. One of the girls who still lived in our home city took more furniture, and so she graciously gave my daughter, who lived in California, the painting of the girl with the balloons and the antique clock. Some siblings draw numbers and take turns sorting through furniture and silver and jewelry; some turn everyone loose with stickers to mark what they each would choose "when the time comes." Some mothers and fathers make lists, in control to the end. After the end. In the will. Some children or grandchildren don't really care. Some families apportion according to need.

Realizing that there is a potential land mine under the living room carpet or in the kitchen cabinets, I really don't want to think now about defusing it. I'm sure it will not explode. It will work itself out, peaceably, I'm sure. Except, perhaps, for the key ring.

Things That Go Bump in the Night

Even for the most sanguine of us — and there aren't very many Pollyannas around these days — there are nights when the demons and monsters gnaw on us. These are real demons in today's world. We have heard the most recent warning that synagogues and Jewish schools might be the next likely terrorist targets — with stolen fuel trucks. (As it is, the doors to our temple have been kept locked since 9/11.) This warning is announced as "uncorroborated . . . not specific." Meant for the eyes and ears of law-enforcement agencies, it ends up on all the TV news reports. On a beautiful summer night, as you turn off the eleven o'clock news and close your eyes, you are not softly humming "In the Good Old Summertime" as your lullaby.

On some days, we have heard unsettling family news. We have personal concerns about our health; we have even more concerns about the health and well-being of friends. The market is tanking. These are all facts that disturb us and can disturb our sleep.

In this state of mind, the imagined demons can run loose. We hear an unfamiliar noise in the house. We wonder if we locked all the doors. Is it possums or squirrels we hear on the roof? It is something — something unfamiliar. It is always two-thirteen a.m. Why is that? It is usually the night of a full moon. I know why that is.

When Bobby was a very little boy, before he could go to sleep at night, we had a ritual. I kissed him good night, turned on the night-light, put a glass of water by his bed, and said, "Ruly and duck and goose and wolf, car, airplane, hoo-hoo and the one who burps, get out of here." I have no recollection of how, together, he and I invented that meaningless list. But it worked and he slept a dreamless, happy sleep. (I might not have blown his cover on this childhood memory, but he admitted it himself in a magazine article.) Other grown children, I feel sure, have good memories of similar comforting rituals. If you really want to get yourself upset, though, think of the thousands of children today who have no one to comfort them, or even care. Or someone who chooses to abuse them instead of cover them with a soft blanket.

At three a.m., I hear my neighbor's sprinkler system go on. It turns off at three-oh-eight. I get up and take a Tylenol, highly recommended by doctors to banish headaches and monsters. Come morning, I am out looking for lucky signs that the day will go well.

Those signs are everywhere. When my morning paper is leaning right against my front door, I believe I am off to a good day. If I need to mail some letters and I walk them up to my mailbox, and Dennis, my mailman of thirty years standing, has not arrived yet, that is a very good omen: my mail will go out and I won't have to hurry to the post office. If I can turn on the faucet in the garage without using a wrench, that bodes well for the afternoon. If I go to the grocery, and Ben and Jerry's chocolate fat-free yogurt with chocolate brownies is on sale, then, how lucky can I be? If I find a parking meter with some time left on it, I figure the stars are in alignment. I even read it as a portent of a good day to come if I just find a parking space! It is even better still if I make it back to the car before my time has expired.

We people of this certain age have had a

lot of years to figure out what is luck, both good and bad, how much control we have over what will happen, how we will feel if the dice roll one way or the other. We seniors have had all these years to know ourselves; still, we cannot predict if we are going to have a night of foreboding or a day of optimism — or a day of foreboding and a peaceful night. Just last evening, at nine-fifteen, I looked at the clock and said, out loud, "Bob, I've got it knocked. I can read for forty-five minutes, watch Aaron Brown, and then go to sleep." There was no time to worry or stew or make a list. I had clear sailing until eleven p.m. and a fine night's sleep.

If we cannot control the minor deities or the devils, then best befriend them. In the wee small hours of the morning, I often recite the twenty-third psalm to myself. In truth, it works a lot better than the Tylenol.

Remember . . .

Almost anything can trigger a memory. It's not *almost* anything, it is *anything:* sights, sounds, days of the week, time of the year, music, a familiar-looking face, a bar of soap. As the years go by, we have accumulated so many memories that it is hard to imagine the brain cells can keep track of them all. They can't or they don't — not all at once. But when called on, they can come like waves, sequentially, one after the other after the other. This happens to me all of the time. I find them a true blessing and a phenom-enon, as they come running out of their hiding places, shouting "Remember when," "Remember where." And I remember:

The Kentucky Derby: When I was in high school, I had a friend whose father knew how to "place a bet." In the mid-nineteen-thirties, offtrack betting was not exactly savory, and it was never quite ex-plained to me how my fifty cents got from me to the bookmaker at the other end of a telephone line, somewhere. I always associate that bet with the smell of lilacs in our yard, where this junior Nathan Detroit and I sat on the front steps, and I handed over the cash. There were no G-men lurking in the bushes, and I never won, so it didn't matter much: it was just so worldly to know a boy who knew a man who knew a bookie! I chose my horse the scientific way a teenager would: I liked the name. I think it was Easy Grades that won some years later, but that was a name I would surely have chosen. Bob and I always watched the annual Derby broadcast, never knowing more as an adult than I did as a girl, until 1963, when Chateaugay, a Columbus horse from the Darby Dan stables, won. Ten years later, I was in a Florida hospital room, watching with my mother, who had just received a pacemaker (not nearly so common then as now); that she could sit up in bed and watch after an endless hospital stay meant that we might come home soon. Secretariat took the roses and went on to win the Triple Crown. To me, it felt like a good omen for my mother. This year, as I sat in front of the TV again, all of those Derbys crowded in on me. I watched the same track, but the jockeys, the horses, and the trainers who, each year, have such an individual and personal story, all sixty-seven of them blurred into one, and it was my story I was remembering. What really pleased me was to see that this year, as Wynton Marsalis played his beautiful trumpet, the revised lyrics to "My Old Kentucky Home" rolled across the screen, so that at long last, the sun was meant to shine bright on all *people*. About time!

The cushions on the deck: We had a lovely screen porch in the house where the children grew up. (I know that "screened" is the proper adjective, but here in the heartland, "screen" is part of the name, hence a noun. Just another curious thing to remember.) We had summer furniture with cushions and we protected it from the rain that might blow in with canvas drops that had to be rolled up or down — depending on the weather forecast. Bob was very meticulous about it; I beat the blowing rain most of the time, but the rattan rug got soaked often enough that it ended, when we moved, in the trash. Thus, I set the scene for the outdoor furniture in this house where I now live.

Our very first home improvement was a stone patio, with a circular bed in the middle, planted with myrtle, to disguise an old tree stump. We brought some redwood furniture from Bryden Road and bought lovely new yellow cushions. So new and lovely (we thought) that at the first sprinkle, the cry went out: "Put the cushions under the overhang!" Gradually, we got older and the furniture did the same; replacement cushions were easier to come by. Water can seep through the new cushions and they dry out — eventually. Sometimes it takes a few days after a really hard rain — which we had with the tornado warning last week. As I lay in bed, listening to the sirens and the amplified voice that said "This is a tornado warning," I thought about the cushions.

I debated with myself whether to stay in my warm, comfortable bed or to go to our lower level, as I knew I should. What was foremost in my mind was not whether I was going to be blown to Oz; my first thought was that Bob would have been out on the deck and down on the patio, bringing the cushions under the overhang. I could literally hear him saying to me "Phyl, it is pouring rain and all of the cushions are still on the furniture!" I decided I ought to go where it was safe, but I felt guilty and lonely — and very sad.

Ivory Soap: I was at a meeting last

week, and before we got down to the business at hand, we chitchatted. It was May and our gardens were on all of our minds. (More about *that* later!) One friend said that someone had told her to put bars of Ivory Soap in the hosta bed to keep the deer from eating the leaves. Reflecting but briefly on the tragedy of urban sprawl sending deer into neighborhoods to forage for food, I leapt in another direction. Who would think that the words "Ivory Soap" would send me on such a journey?

Soap: I learned in elementary school how our pioneering ancestors made soap from fats and lye and water. Like, who cared? Except for Mr. Procter and Mr. Gamble, who would eventually refine Ivory into a household name, and a substantial empire. Fourth grade, 1929: that was a bad year all around.

The family soap of choice was Ivory in the house of my growing up. It was, we were told, 99.44% pure, and we learned for ourselves that it floated, too. Ivory was there in the bathrooms and in my subconscious; it was the only soap to use. (Getting consumers young is not just a myth.)

A few bars of Ivory Soap were in the first grocery bag that, as a bride, I brought to our first home, from the store in Medford, Oregon. Boy, had I made a major mistake! "I hate the smell of Ivory Soap," Bob said. He was serious and he meant it. How was I going to resolve this, I wondered. In our railroad-flat apartment, you walked into the living room, right through the kitchen, and then the bedroom, and then the tiny bathroom. A bar of Ivory in the kitchen, some unknown brand in the bathroom — it wouldn't work. It was imperative that we reach a compromise. And so we compromised: I never bought another bar of Ivory Soap again. You can breathe a sigh of relief, however, Mr. P. and Mr. G.: for years, we drank Folgers coffee, ate Pringles, and brushed with Crest.

March 7: Yesterday, Tim called to tell me that, among other things, they have a new golden retriever puppy. She has been named Cammi for the captain of the United States women's Olympic hockey team, and her birthday is March 7. (She joins two other dogs, three ducks, two guinea pigs — one pregnant — one fish, and five children.) In that maelstrom of activity, the reason Cammi's birthday is important is that March 7 was Bob's birthday, too.

These last three years, that has been a day to go to the cemetery. Before that, it was a major event and a celebration. For Bob's fiftieth, a big party at the country club, with the guests costumed as their favorite stars; for his seventieth, all the children and grandchildren with us in Florida, singing, to "New York, New York," "Start spreading the news/ His day is today/ We've come to be a part of it/ Bob Greene, Bob Greene"; for his eightieth, another Florida party, with the invitation promising a full-service bar to include Alka-Seltzer, bottles of Geritol, aspirin, prune juice, Poli-Grip, Mylanta, and industrial-strength Milk of Magnesia. All of us "snowbirds," dancing and laughing: a happy time.

The last birthday, his eighty-third, is a reminiscence I could do without. We were guests at dinner, seated with a couple who had had too much alcohol. They grew increasingly insulting and unpleasant, until Bob stood up, suggesting to me that we really ought to leave, and the husband snarled, "Do you want to fight?" to my poor, worn husband, too exhausted even to wander around during cocktails. What a final "celebration."

Probably, if Bob could be the one doing

the remembering, he would tell us all about his seventh birthday and his favorite gift ever: a scooter. How proudly he scooted it home from his friend Allen's in the cool, early evening — out after dark, if only just across the street. The stars were shining and the moon was bright, he always told me, becoming once again a thrilled, proud little boy: thrilled to have the gift of his dreams, proud to be seven. It is a pure and lovely little story. There is no ". . . and then someone stole it" or ". . . and then he fell off and scraped his knee." It is the kind of memory we all have tucked away somewhere, that can sustain us at the most unexpected moments.

Delta will no longer have paper tickets: Reading that news article this week proved to me that we are completely in the (bright) new world. No ticket to present at the gate; fly to California on a home-printed e-mail? That is wonderful. That is progress. There is much I do not cheer in this new world of communicating; this I do.

For my sixty-fifth birthday, Bob took me to Boston for a sentimental journey. We stayed at the Copley Hotel, had a drink at the "Merry-Go-Round" bar (which is no longer the "Merry-Go-Round" bar), and then went to have dinner at Locke-Ober (which is still Locke-Ober). Boston is such a well-planned, compact city — we walked from the Commons to Faneuil Hall market to the New England Aquarium and the Old North Church. We rented a car and drove to Wellesley on Sunday afternoon. Packing for home that evening, happy that we had come, Bob checked our tickets and found they were issued for Columbus to Boston.

On our way to Boston, we had handed them the tickets for the return leg — and they had accepted them. (I say "they" and "them" only because I have no idea what airline we were using.) Bob was upset as only Bob could get upset, and made many phone calls, not getting much satisfaction. Of course, we arrived home safely: no one suspected us of stealing the tickets; there was no hassle at the gate. It is even a rather pointless tale to tell, except that the small notice about Delta triggered all of this — in one quick glance at the newspaper.

Open and Shut

Opening your life to new experiences is easy. One of the best pieces of advice I got as a new widow was to try everything at least once. Take an out-of-town trip if you have the chance. Go to Machu Picchu if you are able. Havana is allowing more tourists in. Rent a house in Provence, a castle in Spain. That is all hyperbole, sure, but don't refuse an invitation to a lunch or a dinner or a bridge game! Go along with the group when they buy tickets to a show or a concert. It is a surefire way to open up your world — your whole world!

Then, pray tell, why is it so damn hard to open a jar, a can, a package, or shrink-wrap? Your world, yes; a bottle of aspirin, no way! I use "damn" in this context as a publishable expletive; just struggle with removing five Post-it pads from a package that encases them in heavy plastic bonded to the edges of a piece of cardboard. As I search for scissors, a letter opener, and needle-nose pliers (no place to grab the cardboard edges!), I am muttering a lot worse than "damn" to myself.

One of the sadder truths about aging, and one that came as a great surprise, is how much strength we lose in our hands without realizing it. We may avoid the gym and workouts in front of the TV, or even the mandatory walk three times a week. Like it or not, though, we use our hands continually, even while bypassing all those other exertions. Everyone understands the phrase "Let your fingers do the walking": they exercise; we sit. We feel pretty sprightly; they can hardly perform. 'Tis a mystery.

There are all sorts of gadgets that should help. Cheapest, simplest, often given away by banks and dry cleaners, is the flat rubber disc — with the imprinted logo. Is that good or bad PR for the giver of the gift, if the jar refuses to be opened? There are many variations of the metal device that can accommodate many sizes of snap-tight or screw-on lids. Fitting the opener to the lid is not too difficult; to turn the handle or the vise-like grips takes us back to the basic problem — we don't have the strength to do it.

I remember precisely the moment in 1982 when the demand for safe packaging became urgent and inevitable. Our number-two granddaughter was three months old, and her mother had brought her to Columbus to visit both sets of grandparents. I decided to let all the friends and relatives come to our house at one time to admire her, and had invited them for tea. (No watercress sandwiches; Coca-Cola and cookies, I think.) She was all dressed up, lying on Bob's handsome bedspread, and I was getting myself be-lipsticked. We had been in this house for ten years, and had just splurged on redecorating the bedroom, the previous owners' velvet swaths not being really "me." It was around three in the afternoon when the phone rang. "Don't take any Tylenol!" Bobby told me. "Seven people have died who took Tylenol in the last few days. Some bottles are contaminated." Thus I shall always remember the date, because the granddaughter is now twenty — and so, then, is the decor of the bedroom.

Of course, it is wonderful that products are "tamperproof," but that you need a chain and tackle to open a can of coffee, a carving knife to disengage the locking plastic from the bottle top on a half gallon of milk, or a man with a large pair of pliers to pull the tab on a padded manila envelope, does seem a little overboard.

One sick and demented human being, never found, has changed the way we put items in boxes, bottles, and envelopes. The accompanying cost in research and development, and packaging, has been, of course, passed along to the consumer. How well we know, after 9/11, that safety — whether in the skies or in the drugstore — is expensive.

And I have not even mentioned wine bottles. Corkscrews can, at times, partially uncork. In extremis, however, I have clamped the half-pulled cork in my back teeth which, to date, have not aged as rapidly as my previously powerful paws — thank heavens. Talk about opening up the world: all I want is an occasional glass of chardonnay!

The Gumble Chip

Eliza Gumble and Aaron Harmon, my father's parents, were married on November 27, 1884 in Columbus, Ohio. Their very large families had emigrated from Bavaria in the early 1850s and, as recorded in the 1880 census, ten family members lived in the household of the first generation of American Harmons and nine in the Gumbles'. Also, Molly Harmon, Aaron's sister, married Henry Gumble, Eliza's brother, making our gene pool deep and wide.

The Gumble and Harmon names, as such, are vanishing. There are no Gumble men, and my brother's four-year-old grandson is our last chance to preserve the Harmons. (We had a cousin who seriously considered changing his last name to Gumble, but he had three children of his own and it seemed an empty gesture.) Yet, what with all the begettings that followed that 1884 marriage, six generations later there are innumerable fifth cousins and some seventh, many of whom do not know each other at all — even their names.

Being a sentimentalist, not a geneticist, when I see familiar traits (i.e., peculiarities) in any member of this far-flung clan, I joyfully say, "Aha! the Gumble chip." I unscientifically attribute the gene to the Gumble DNA because the Gumbles kept having more progeny after that first generation, but much of our shared similarities are Harmon-based, I am sure.

It was as a girl that I first became aware of this peculiar (almost) abnormality. When my brother was young, but old enough to play outside without constant supervision — remember, we are talking the early thirties here — every time my father would hear a car brake, he would rush to the window to check on the whereabouts of his young son. I never noticed any other fathers doing that when I was at their house. That was a very Gumble chip response in a Harmon man.

A minor distinction (having nothing to do with worry, actually), is that Gumbles have their very own inflections for certain words and phrases. "Idea" puts the emphasis definitely on the "I," and when a person is "ten years old," it's the years that are accented. There were some forty families in Columbus in 1880 who had lived in the community of Mittlesinn, in the southeastern section of old Germany, and I have never heard any of their descendants use that distinctive pronunciation. When you hear those cadences, ease into any subject that might alarm the listener: a member of the Gumble clan is in the crowd.

According to the historians, we began in this new country of ours as shopkeepers. The patriarch of the Harmons ran a grocery; of the Gumbles, a saloon. There are a lot of store clerks in our early backgrounds — so when did the theater bug get into our heritage? My cousin Henny, Henry and Molly's granddaughter, put the notion in my head that it all might have something to do with the Columbus water!

We have a bona fide star of TV and stage; two fairly well-known actors, a young woman who works in casting, and two up-and-coming young actors who are single-purposed in the direction they are heading. And those are only the ones of whom I am reasonably sure. A handful of them are in Hollywood and have not met.

It is the Gumble worry-chip, nevertheless, that does set us apart. My daughter says it is implanted in our butts, which is as good a place as any. We all have it; not every specific worry in every Gumble/

Harmon, but every one of us has this unique G-chip capable of producing any number of worries, at any given time. All kinds of people worry about some things some of the time. We just w-o-r-r-y!

These are the questions (large and small) that the Gumble worry-chip produces: have I made enough salad for my mahjong game? Will my granddaughter be happy at the college she has chosen? Should I let my son with the brand-new driver's license use the car? How reliable is the baby-sitter? How will my MRI turn out? Do these shoes match this purse? Why isn't my son home yet? How wise is it to go to Europe now? Will I be invited to the wedding? What can I do about my bunions? (That is a family-wide worry.) Did the fish in that restaurant taste kind of funny? Why are they asking me to have another mammogram? Did I choose the best or just the cheapest roofer? (How can they be one and the same?) Is that nagging pain only indigestion? Why hasn't X called this week? Will India or Pakistan use any of their nuclear arsenal? I'm afraid I've chosen the wrong driveway resealer. I have no i-dea what I should wear to the meeting. Did I remember to take my morning medicines? Will my hospitalization cover that? If I invite R, do I have to invite S and T? I'm eighty-two *years* old, why am I worrying about any of this?

How Does Your Garden Grow?

Not at all — not the petunias nor the impatiens nor the begonias. Not this year nor last year nor the year before that. I keep having "issues" — that wonderful new buzz-word — issues with the soil and the mulch, and a whole slew of gardeners. In the last few years, since the death of my husband, my heart has not been in my gardening and, obviously, neither have my hands.

I should have developed some aptitude for gardening. When I was a little girl, I used to follow my mother around as we cut huge bouquets of larkspur and snap-dragons and dahlias. I even have an old snapshot of us together, her arms full of the bounty of our backyard. What I did inherit from her good genes was very strong teeth; from her not-so-good, I have heart problems and horrible feet. From whence came the beds barren of blooms?

When we moved to this house thirty years ago, three middle-aged sisters lived in the house in back of us. They were single — widowed or never married. One ran a pharmacy, one was a professor, and one had been, among other occupations, an executive secretary. We always referred to them as "the ladies," as in, "The ladies' flowers look beautiful this year." They all had green thumbs and a gorgeous yard. Our house is atop a sloping lawn that runs down to what is laughingly called a creek; their lawn ran up from the creek to their rambling house and, all around and up and down, they had beds and beds of magnificent plantings. As the years went by, the planted beds grew fewer. First, the professor died; then, the pharmacist. Sarah was alone in the house and there were no flower beds — just planters around the driveway up top. Then she sold the house and moved to an apartment building.

We got new neighbors, who had a nice garden; it just wasn't "the ladies'." The upside to this story is that I don't feel quite as obsessed about keeping-up-with-the-neighbors. At this writing, however, I am running in last place, and it is the last lap — the first week in May. I haven't even bought my annuals. I'm not sure what to buy to put where, but I am casting a wide net for someone to step up to the shovel — and dig, dig, dig.

A friend of my daughter's is an amateur

gardener. I say "amateur" only to distinguish her from someone who gets paid to do this work for others — she does it for herself and her house. I am sure that to her neighbors, she becomes the homeowner with the awesome plantings; she is her neighborhood's "lady." One late afternoon, she and DG came over to commiserate with and advise me. It was like all other May evenings this year: cold, damp, drizzling. As we walked around my yard, I kept making notes in my steno notebook. She said things like yucca, miscanthus, grasses, and splitting daylilies. I said, "Let's go in and have a glass of wine and order a pizza." This was the moment I needed to ask her to find me someone to take over — a professional; professional gardener. Shortly thereafter, such a wonder-worker appeared, took the same garden walk, mapped out a plan, and promised to return with the return of the sunshine. The world and I are still waiting.

This May it is too wet and cold to dig — or even walk in the yard. It has rained some eighty-five percent of the month; it hasn't just rained, it has stormed. Some nights I ignore the tornado warnings that only run across the TV screen; it seemed wise to respond the night the sirens went off at four a.m. and the loudspeakers were blaring, "Go to a safe place immediately." As I headed for our lower level, it seemed I ought to do something useful downstairs, something to help me pass the time. Earlier that evening, I had bought a new screwlike device that would hold together the two little knobs that you use to open the screen door to the deck. I had even taken the old, stripped screw with me to the hardware store to be sure the length was correct. When I got home, I found that, of course, it was not. So on my way down the stairs, I took the knobs with me, remembering that Bob had a toolbox down there with a variety of nails, tacks, screws, bolts — everything. That was the hardware I should have "shopped" first; I had wasted seven cents and had missed a TV show I wanted to see just to avoid the stairs! Once down, though, I began to go through each well-organized compartment and, sure enough, I found just what I needed. The all-clear sounded; I went back to bed. The next morning, the screen door was back in working order.

It was either that storm, or the one before it, or the other bad one after it, that made the ground too wet to hold the roots of the "junk" tree just beyond the pool fence. On a Sunday, I noticed that the tree was leaning precariously over the fence, veering toward the pool at a dangerously low angle. First thing Monday morning, I called Davey Tree. They have been in the tree business so long that they don't even need a display ad in the yellow pages; Martin Davey Sr. was governor of Ohio from 1934 to 1938, and, in fact, he and Bob's mother had dated when they both were at Oberlin, in college. We have seldom called anyone else for our tree problems, which have not been minimal.

They promised to come out Wednesday to take a look. Monday evening, as I was locking the door to the deck, I saw the entire tree down on the pool, in all its junk-y glory: vines, leaves, poison ivy, and its entire trunk. Tuesday morning early, I called Davey to tell them, "Forget the estimate, come get the tree" — which they did by the next Wednesday. On the bill, which was just slightly less than my insurance deductible, I noticed that they had upgraded the tree from junk to cherry. What I needed back there along the creek bank was a latter-day George Washington; an ex-president for my tree instead of an ex-governor.

If the tree fell silently on the pool — and

the pool cover and the fence — and no-body heard it, I can still vouch that it fell. We are, however, making progress. I can open the screen door to get to the deck; soon the cushions should dry out. Even though I cannot sit out there, I can stand and see that, humbug as I feel about the yard, all the rain has made the bushes, the grass, and even the weeds verdant, lush, and lovely. I am content to wait. I will, eventually, have a garden. I think. I hope.

Aging Appropriately

While I stand by my guns that I continue to feel younger, certainly not every senior citizen feels the same way. (I wish there were a better term than "senior citizen" to describe us. Other choices are worse — oldster, gray panther, golden-ager; in Ohio, we are Golden Buckeyes, with an ID card to prove it. Even the careful, euphemistic AARP magazine title does not quite cut it with *Modern Maturity*.) Those who are well, active, and busy recognize that at any time the tide could turn. It's that very true truism: I'd rather be young and well than sick and old.

We know that we cannot look as young as we once did. If we care enough, there are face-lifts and now Botox — but do they really help? Bob always used travel as his metaphor for the "aging" look — as in, "She's got a lot of miles on her." (And, yes, it usually was a she to whom he was referring.)

I am ashamed to say that I am a little offended each time someone pulls open a heavy door for me — at the grocery, the doctor's office, or the library. I am appreciative, of course, because those doors all take a lot of energy, and I always say a sincere "thank you." I might not even have gotten in or out without the help. Politeness like that in today's society is rare and wonderful. It is just a deep-down hurt that I am unable to do it easily by myself, and that the "lot of miles on her" say to a kind stranger: "Give this old gal a helping hand." (The helping hand is so often that of another old gal. Darn it.)

A contemporary of mine still golfs three times a week; her regular partners are all much younger than she (probably most of the golfers at her course are younger); kindly, after they all finish putting, one of the other three automatically picks the flag up from the green and replaces it in the hole. My contemporary is an amazingly active woman, and she feels a little diminished — a little deflated — because she knows her own capabilities, and replacing the pin is one of them. At the same time, she is especially fond of her friends as they do this for her. Wounded pride is an exceedingly complicated emotion when it is kindness that wounds.

I had a very thoughtful e-mail from a *Moonglow* reader who is finding "the subtle, but real downgrading of my place in society. Old ladies are not highly valued in our society today. They are treated with courtesy but with little interest. . . . My life contribution as wife, mother, and the nurturer of two-and-a-half complete families seems largely irrelevant to the world. I still draw on my seven years as a teacher and three years as an office manager when I need to command respect from people who do not know me."

These thoughts have been simmering on my back burner. At what stage do older people become irrelevant and somewhat marginalized? Is it when they cannot walk fast enough, remember long enough, participate often enough, or think well enough? If asked how we are doing, we shed our years when we are able to check that we can do all of the above. Some of it is within our power. Not all. Once you are "of a certain age," there is always the nagging feeling that, along with the respect, there is an undercurrent of condescension or of being a little patronized. We may desire to stay relevant, but life is hurrying by and there is so much to process!

Last week, there was an article about staying "hip." It began: "The fifty-year-old first realized he was no longer hip when he quit checking *Rolling Stone*'s list of top albums on college campuses." What if you are of such an age that you never, ever understood *Rolling Stone* the few times you saw it? You already are way beyond unhipness, just as you are way beyond fifty. The article was headlined: "Broken Hip." So comforting. There was an instructive sidebar to help you feel updated, not so "five minutes ago," with a list of "Then . . . and Now." Then — *The Jeffersons*, now — *The Bernie Mac Show*; then — Blondie, now — Pink; then — George Clooney, now — Josh Hartnett; etc.; etc.; etc. I hardly recognized a "now." I even had trouble with a few of the "thens."

As we age, one of the pluses is that we don't have to be "with it." The minus: if we are not with it, we are "without it"; we are marginalized. We find ourselves to be "has-been" names when organizations are developing sponsor lists for events. We need to fight the tendency to urge a church group, with which we are working, that "that is the way we always did it." If we are wise, we weigh our words a little more carefully, lest we become rambling windbags. We don't want to be contentious. The trick is to stay young enough to be an asset while accepting the "subtle and real

downgrading of our place in society." So
says my e-mail friend.

In our Longboat Key years, Joan and
Betty and I often turned up on the beach
with the same bathing suit — attractive, la-
dylike. Called "swim dresses" by Elizabeth
Stewart, who manufactured them, they
were designed for women who needed the
skirt and the separate panties. Was it because the bathing suits were age-
appropriate that we found we were compatible in many other ways? Probably not,
but our beach-walking wardrobe sent up
the first flare.

This is a great time of life, and a time to
be proactive. Staying in the center of
things helps avoid the margins. We can remain in that mainstream, if we remember
to wear a swim dress and not think we can
still turn heads in a bikini.

How Old Is Old?

I just caught the last few minutes of the local evening news, when I heard something about "young at heart." Hm, I thought. That's probably another good euphemism for "senior citizen," a word problem I had been thinking about for a few days. Admiring but condescending, it resonated under my not-so-thin skin.

The story was about a group of seventy-and-over softball players. We are big on softball players here in the heartland, so it didn't seem to warrant more of a story on the news than it was getting.

In the next morning's paper, it was right in the middle of the front page, with two pictures in color. "The Boys of Late Summer" read the headline. (Also reported on page one: the "minor" stories of the White House response to criticism of the president's handling of what he knew and when he knew it before 9/11, of the body that was found in Karachi undoubtedly being that of Daniel Pearl, and of fifteen hundred workers being moved out of downtown to the suburbs.)

Why this softball league of six teams, all with players over seventy, is news is that it is the only league of its kind in the nation's cold-weather states. There are only a few elsewhere — Florida, California, Arizona. For more than a decade, fifty-and-over and sixty-and-over leagues have been sprouting up. Now, the sixty-pluses are turning seventy, and they still want to play. Same time next year, watch for the eighty-and-overs. There's a seventy-seven-year-old shortstop out there, and in three years he won't want to be benched. I also know a man who plays tennis in the ninety-and-over USTA-sponsored national championships. I do know a little more about tennis than slow-pitch softball, and I understand why the preference of this senior group is clay courts: the game is hard enough on the body without the playing surface being really hard, too. Maybe they should aim for the grass at Wimbledon.

Baseball is not necessarily my sport, but young-at-heart is my motivation. Each spring, I am invited to the Columbus Foundation for a series of three lecture-and-lunches; it is a way to stay in touch, to learn more about what is going on, to see others as interested in the community as I am. My day that had begun with a news-paper article about a game on grass and dirt had, by noon, put me in space: John Glenn, born July 18, 1921, was the speaker; his subject was The John Glenn Institute for Public Service and Public Policy, a project that is getting underway at The Ohio State University. The Institute's purpose is to involve young people in civic issues and to promote leadership qualities in the generations to come.

John Glenn first flew the Mercury space-ship in February, 1962. He returned to space in 1998, participating in experiments to determine how space affects young bodies much in the same way nature does aging, earthbound bodies. Senator Glenn was seventy-seven on that second flight. He is eighty as he accepts yet another chal-lenge. Good for him. Good for anybody who claims new territory or cedes none of the old.

Keith Richards is fifty-nine and he could be the grandfather of Britney Spears or the Back Street Boys, yet it is the Rolling Stones who are getting three hundred dol-lars for some tickets on their new concert tour. So we "young at heart" have all the heart we need to participate in any number of ways and in any number of venues.

We all know the "well-known" senior citizens: Grandma Moses, the Delaney sisters, Georgia O'Keeffe, Studs Terkel, and the pope. But who, Fred Rogers used to ask, are the people in your neighborhood, the people you see each day? They are the men who help you carry out your groceries, the women who greet you at Wal-Mart, the pink ladies in the hospitals — contemporaries of Studs and Georgia and the pope. All participants.

I must admit, however, that quite recently I saw a headline that made me say aloud, "Good heavens, this is too, too much." What I was reading was that "Age needn't limit distance runner, coach says." Since my (tongue-in-cheek) motto is "Never stand when you can sit, never sit when you can lie," I was much relieved to find that the article was about people in their fifties.

Reborn on the Fourth of July

It was almost ten minutes of ten when the Bexley police car came down Roosevelt Avenue, leading the Bexley Celebrations Association's forty-third annual Independence Day parade. They had left the Maryland Avenue school at precisely nine-thirty, and the police car was followed by thirty-six antique cars and trucks carrying the reuning classes of 1977, 1982, 1987, 1992, and 1997, and by convertibles with Mayor David Madison, Citizen of the Year Chris Masoner, the members of City Council (at least those who were in town), and the superintendent of schools. Car #31 received the most applause of all: "Rubino's: A Bexley Tradition." That is what it said on the sign — but no one needed the sign because Tommy and Frank, in person — Rubino's CEOs and master pizza-makers — were there, riding in the back seat. The Ali Baba Temple minicars, the color guard of the Jewish war veterans, the Baha'i community of Bexley (carrying a banner), the Bexley High School marching band, the Bexley Boosters and team captains, and the decorated bicycles and tricycles came marching along in the ninety-eight-degree heat. (The first July after Bob died, a uniformed group from the Bexley American Legion Post #430 marched by and, blindsided completely, I burst into unexpected tears.) This year, Tim, standing beside me, said to his sixteen-year-old son, Tucker, "Son, I have two words for you — Hartley cheerleaders," and I knew I was right where I belonged: on the parade route for the forty-third time.

When we lived in Bexley, we lived four houses east of the parade route, so our corner was Bryden and Roosevelt. Our next-door neighbor was in the automotive parts business and owned an old fire engine. One year, our children got to ride in it and activate the siren. Have the world champion Yankees ever had a more triumphal ride down Broadway? Then, we moved to the house I live in now, and we had to drive in to the parade. First, Tim lived right where the parade began, and when he moved to Colorado, we congregated at my brother and sister-in-law's, where tables set up in their garage offer Bloody Marys and red, white, and blue donuts and soft drinks of every kind. Literally hundreds of people stop by to say hello, greet old friends (you know you know them — but what is their name?) and feel the kind of patriotism that does flourish in the heartland of the free and the home of the brave.

There is a sentence atop the printed program that says, "Please stand when the flag passes by your viewing area." I was pretty strict about enforcing that rule when the children were little and sitting on the curb. Now, people are milling about and standing, and there is no time to sit down and get up again between flags. Yet, when a marching band does come by, playing "The Stars and Stripes Forever," no one needs to be told what to do.

I love the Fourth of July; it is the perfect time for a family reunion. I'm of a mindset that says bratwurst and potato salad are tastier than turkey and dressing, or pork and sauerkraut, or ham and scalloped potatoes. It is the calendar date I always anticipate. Our reunions don't always work out or come to pass. We don't get everybody here every year, but I remember them cumulatively, and in my mind I paint my own picture of everyone here on every Fourth.

This was a good year — not a hundred percent attendance, but a lot of activity,

Rubino's pizza three times in one short week (four, if you count zapping a few pieces of leftovers in the microwave after the fireworks), and all of my brother and SIL's (that's book-group shorthand for sister-in-law) children and grandchildren for swimming and a picnic. DG and her Martha's Vineyard, lifelong friend Marcia, who is living in Columbus for the summer, really took over the hostessing and did all the hard work, while I just enjoyed! Enjoyed!

Even if I could convene every single one of my family, Bob would still be absent. That is one piece of the family picture that will forever keep the painting incomplete.

On Friday, I took Tim, Tuck, and Hannah to the airport. As Tim hugged me, I felt that familiar tickling feeling in my nose, and knew that tears would soon follow. I did only a fair job of maintaining as they walked to the outdoor check-in counter. I knew I hadn't fooled them at all. Anti-climax: I couldn't get the car in gear; it was stuck on "park." Hannah was watching. I motioned her over, and she motioned for Tucker, who asked, "Have you turned the motor on, Wede?" — and then I could laugh at myself, and they could walk in to the airport. The end of a happy visit on a very high note.

Reborn, reenergized, reunited on the Fourth of July. Hooray for those Founding Fathers who allowed us, at least for one day of the year, to be Yankee Doodle Dandies.

The Changing City

My city is no different from most other cities. It once was a small, easily traversed grid of downtown streets; the sparsely populated residential neighborhoods were located not very far outside that central area. It has now grown outward in all directions; it has grown to be different in each direction. We have seen gentrification in some older neighborhoods; we have seen some older neighborhoods become home to the urban poor. We have sprawling suburbs and, out beyond them, the exurbs. We have shelves full of master plans for orderly growth. We have growth fueled by developers (my daughter calls all of those new housing complexes "twirls" — the streets that wind in and out and around and back into each other). We have whole communities spring up almost overnight: shopping malls, housing, offices, hotels, and golf courses. It is quite incredible to have watched this, almost from the beginning, and to marvel at the changes.

The east side of town was always our family locale. Twenty-five-or-so years ago, on a nice sunny day, I drove my aunt and mother out to see what was happening farther east still. It was a modest growth: an enclosed mall with a branch of our downtown department store, a movie theater, a restaurant, some small shops, a card shop, and some shoe stores. (A "branch" store was quite a revolutionary idea then. If you wanted to shop, you were expected to go *downtown*.) "Oh," said my aunt, plaintively, "I wish things wouldn't change so much. I loved it so the way it was."

I was thinking of that last evening, when I was invited to an elegant restaurant in the gigantic building that is home to our first major-league sports team: the Columbus Blue Jackets. Right downtown, we have an entire new district, the Arena District. Hockey season having ended, it was reasonably quiet but, nevertheless, awesome. There are two gigantic rinks (one for practice). This is maintenance season: new logos for new sponsors were being stenciled onto the surface before the new layer of ice is to be put down. Seventeen-thousand square feet is devoted to restaurants in that building alone. In the surrounding buildings: more restaurants, offices, parking lots, and a brand new movie theater.

The entire project is, in fact, in the very downtown I knew as a child. The arch from our old Union Station — the train station I left from to go to camp and to college — has been preserved. A lovely green allee runs behind it, shrubs and trees on either side, and benches where you can sit and enjoy your memories of yesterday and imagine your tomorrow.

"But where are we, exactly?" I had to ask. "Where did all of this come from?" Even though I had read about it, seen it from a distance, and even felt kind of chauvinistic about the Blue Jackets, I was disoriented. Where I was, it turns out, was on the site of the old Ohio State Penitentiary, an ancient, gray, stone pile I must have passed three hundred times during the course of my life — or more. This was a route we once used to go to the football stadium or to the Olentangy River Road to head north. This piece of the city was always clear in my mind's eye. It is now something completely different.

The Pen was an institution with a dreadful history, recounted by David Lore in the *Columbus Dispatch* in a long article, written as the Pen's obituary in 1984, when it was closed down. Three hundred and fifteen men and women died in its electric chair; many more on its gallows and in its torture chambers before that. "There are no ghosts in the histories, the stories, the memories of the place," Lore wrote. "Even ghosts, it would seem, don't care to tarry on Spring Street one moment more than necessary."

But real people are there now: O. Henry, "Bugsy" Moran, Sam Sheppard have been replaced by the hockey fans, the drinkers, the moviegoers, and the diners who prefer "pan-roasted venison with ragout of morels" or "Fuyu persimmon, tangerine salad with Cambazola and candied pecans" to "cornbread, bacon and beans . . . served on 'rust-eaten tin plates.' " It is chilling to be on that spot and know what horrors existed in our very midst.

Of the landmarks we destroy, there are hundreds, thousands worth saving; many, like the old Pen, need to be demolished. Ours is a city with some visionary leadership; an outdated, outmoded prison has given way to a visionary regeneration. As goes this city, so goes the whole country. What I wish is that I could take a peek at it all in the twenty-second century!

Four Funerals and a Wedding

When Hugh Grant and Andie MacDowell kept running into each other at one event after another (four weddings, one funeral), it was a light and frothy movie; in the past month, my close encounters of the wrong kind have shifted the balance and changed the ratio, converting fantasy to reality (four funerals and a wedding — upcoming). At the time — 1994 — I thought the movie was a little callous and, of course, beyond my cultural ken. I am not sure how Ebert and Roeper would judge this real-life version, were it to appear on film; but, strangely enough, I would give it a thumbs-up and even a few stars.

These reflections are, like the movie, not really about the funerals themselves. Needless to say, the funerals were all sad, and the loss felt by the families was devastating to the friends, as well. We all attend such services to grieve with the family, grieve for ourselves, and think about our own mortality. The experts tell us this is so, over and over. They are correct. It is true.

But something wonderful happened after the last service that made me realize how life, friendship, and memories continue on, how sustained and enriched we can be even on the darkest of days. The service I had just attended was for my neighbor, who lived across the street from us when the children were growing up. We went back to that house after the service, to see the family, to pay our respects, and to remember. We talked about Mo driving the Sunday-school carpool, and about the boys who gathered in front of the house every day after school to visit with Lois. DG and Diane stood on the spot in the kitchen where they had always played jacks. This was a condolence call, but it was life-affirming. Rose was almost ninety when she died (we remembered that Mo called her "Ro"), and her long life had been good.

Then, when we walked outside to leave, I found myself standing on the stoop of 2721 Bryden Road, looking across the street at 2722, our old house. All of the owners who followed us — and there have been at least four — have done right by the old place: it looked perfect to me. All up and down the block looked perfect: the grass was cut; the late afternoon sun was shining; and I stood there and recited the name of every single family that had lived in every single house, from Roosevelt to Gould. (Except for one new house that had been built just to the east of ours. When we lived there, it was an open lot owned by our next-door neighbor, turned each summer into a miniature farm with corn and beans and tomatoes; the farmer was a biochemist with a very green thumb, who was generous with his produce. He was so patient in teaching me how to sucker tomatoes, I have been trying ever since.)

I felt an amazing sense of joy in the memories rushing through my mind: running down the street to meet the mailman to get Bobby's first letters from camp; pushing Tim's Taylor Tot to walk with June and Linda; Nippy jumping with excitement and biting Debby's arm in the process. This was a great movie scene; this was *The Best Years of Our Lives* — glowing, warm, and belonging to me forever!

Now I can contemplate the wedding planned for April. It will be in California where the bride and groom live and work. Maggie is my first grandchild, a sophisticated Hollywood person. She has picked out her wedding dress, and the glamorous wedding locale. She has a career. She has a profession. I can anticipate the in-drawn breaths as this beautiful young woman comes down the aisle — and I will see a four-year-old, jumping on the bed yelling, "Wee-Dee, Wee-Dee," the urgency of the call reflecting the urgency of the need: "Come and play Barbies."

I never was very good at that game. The way we played it was that we each took a doll, sat on the floor, and walked the doll around as we (Barbies) talked to each other in a falsetto voice; even Ken was more soprano than baritone. The conversation centered around where we should go: would it be the zoo or the park, or shopping? Shopping usually won, and off we would go to Kmart — a real, thriving Kmart, where Barbie's pony or new dress or tiny accessories were available. Twenty-odd years ago, I did not relish the game; the actual shopping called for the patience of a saint while a discriminating five-year-old chose between the pony with the pink halter and the one with the blue. Today, in retrospect, the panorama down that toy aisle was more beautiful than the Champs-Elysées. And that is the aisle I will be seeing as Maggie walks, on her father's arm, to meet her groom. Who gives this woman, this child? Her parents and her Wee-Dee.

Decision Time . . . or Not

We have been in this place before. "We" being me and you, my readers, deciding along with me, for yourselves, or for me. This may be time to call in a pollster. The old quandary about moving has reared its ugly head "one more once," as Satchmo used to say.

I had an invitation to hear a presentation about a new retirement community that is in the planning/promoting stages. There were to be three such events, and one of them was at a country club very near my house, at a most convenient time. The facility itself looks very nice — lovely, in fact; housing choices range from a studio apartment to a "villa" with two bedrooms, a den, and a garage. The amenities look up-to-the-minute and the financial arrangements seem well-thought-out, with varying options. The great plus is that when the time comes that you must move from "independent" living to "assisted" living (in comfortable quarters), your monthly fee remains the same, guaranteeing you skilled nursing care at no additional cost.

Quite a few friends of long standing showed up; some had even signed up and had made a deposit on the unit of their choice. This is the very kind of place that I had been saying didn't exist in my little corner of Ohio, and here it is, just where I would choose it to be: not much farther east of Debby than I am now currently west. Why am I dragging my feet? Why can't I make up my mind? Haven't I always been decisive? Give me a coin and let me toss it. Let me shoot some dice.

There are a few nights like tonight when I feel sorry — not exactly sorry for myself; just sorry. Turning on the hose is too much; going down the stairs to get to the hose is too much; trying to sprinkle my expensive planting is too much. I have been saying this now for three years. What should I do? Yet, tomorrow, I know I will feel differently, and somehow or other I will do the watering, and somehow or other it will be fall.

A reader had written me about having to give up her home and move to an apartment. It was a place where no animals were allowed, so not only did she lose a beloved home but a beloved dog, too. She was in mourning, again. Her sorrow jumped off the page.

Choices born of necessity are the worst kind; choices fueled by emotion are bad, too. We probably all should be completely rational and do a force-field analysis of the pluses and minuses of all of our decisions. We do not have to abandon a pet to feel bereft — there is always something to miss: the very complicated way to back up the driveway; the small spot in the lawn where there once was a tree stump and is now a declivity that the mower always misses; the particular sound of the plumbing; the view from the bedroom window; the nonbearing apple trees by the pool; the albino squirrel family that has lived in the yard for thirty years. Is this the same squirrel or the grandchild of squirrel #1? Would new owners feed the finches their Nigerian thistle? Would they understand the thermostat? or the dryer vent? How long would it take another tenant to recognize that there is a very unique sound that tells you water is running somewhere in the house? Would the house miss me as I would miss it? How would it fare without my careful stewardship?

When Bobby left for college — he wouldn't be "Bob" for some years to come — the night before he went to Northwestern, he got up from dinner, patted the table, and said, "Well, old table." That was all: just, "Well" — as he patted it twice — "old table." How often I have thought of that over the years, as he has sat down at the same table for another meal. I doubt that the dining room furniture would move with me. Can I pat this house and say, "Well, old house?" This is a question I cannot, cannot answer.

My mind is clear; my crystal ball is not. If I could see as far as 2003, when this project will be ready for occupancy, then I could see myself in the years ahead. If I am blessed enough to keep aging backward, then where I choose to live will be of not much import. I shall likely go through this exercise again and again, weighing options and vacillating and preaching my message only to myself and for myself.

With Edith Wharton nudging me and lobbying me to be "interested in big things, and happy in small ways," it probably doesn't matter where you live but how you live. Persevere with joy.

Filofax Forever

As soon as I opened the package, I knew it was the one thing I had always wanted, and that I hadn't had the sense to realize it. But Susan did; she sent me a maroon, leather Filofax, with pages for names and addresses, pages for notes, twenty "don't forget" pages (with a space for twenty-four "to-dos" on each), lined pages, yellow-paper pages, and a horizontal year calendar — for the year 1989. It was everything my tidy little mind loved. It spoke to the me that liked office-supply stores better than any other retail establishment, except maybe "Blooming-dale's," which was stamped inside the front cover of this book. So there it was — all in one package — and I went right to work.

I transferred all my names and addresses from another book — that had a checked cover and the outline of a woman and some pearls on it (a[d] dress book — get it?) — into this businesslike, six-hole-punch model that would, I knew, serve me well for years to come. Thirteen years later, it is still by my chair, by my phone; it goes where I go if I leave the city. It holds not only the addresses but the earlier-mentioned Christmas lists, plus some financial information and social security numbers and . . . a lot more — a lot.

When I entered the names and addresses in pencil, they were as close to alphabetical order as possible. The tabbed pages indicated two letters each and, in the beginning, the "A's" preceded the "B's." The "A's" were not precisely alphabetical, but I could find whomever I was looking for in a second. As the years went by and I added names (and erased a few), I ran out of spaces in all the sections. I tended to write between addresses; at times, separating the name and address from the phone number by squeezing in another name. Then I took to clipping business cards onto the closest initial, or putting Post-it notes on facing pages. I seldom erased a business name and address even if there was no likelihood that I would ever call them again. I kept the name of a window washer even after he told me he no longer did that kind of work.

One afternoon, about five years ago, I was out, and Bob needed to look for a number. When I got home, I found that he had made a "Danger! Keep Out!" sign and taped it to the cover of the book. He told me that he had gone out and bought me a gift, and what a gift it was: one of those elegant planners that opened out three ways; not only were there pages for names and addresses, but short and long-range plans, meeting notes, and profits and losses. If I had been the president of General Motors, it would have been adequate. Probably the president of Enron should have owned one. Even I might have used some of it when I was more active in the community; it was too much for a retired housewife, and I reluctantly returned it — and vowed to clean up my Filofax. Of course, I never did. I subtracted little; I added everything. It was so full of clipped-on business cards that it would barely close. Plus, all kinds of people had e-mail addresses and fax numbers with which I had to deal.

Last week, I decided to turn over a new leaf; rather, I decided to add new leaves, and bought replacement pages. I started at "A" and began the alphabet once again. It became a very tedious and somber job. I made it through the "I's" reasonably well. There were few of them, and I had earlier erased a few that were heart-rending. Every letter has held some pain:

names of friends who are gone.

I have been proceeding conscientiously. Today, I got to the "J's" and the "K's" and, one right after the other, I had to delete two long-standing entries. The boy whose fraternity pin I had worn all through college had, over the years, been an entry as Mr. and Mrs. in Scarsdale, then in Palm Beach, then he alone at a retirement community in Florida, and finally in a convalescent home in Seattle. He died last December. I could obliterate his name, not the memories. Also, the Jacobson's store that had opened in Columbus, with much fanfare, ten years ago — at our highly anticipated City Center — closed this spring. (City Center itself is not very healthy. We have shopping malls all around the perimeter of the city, pushing ever outward.) I no longer have need for that telephone number or the business cards of the many salespeople, clipped to the page.

I go on to a friend, a "K," who has moved from Columbus to a retirement community in another city, to be near her daughter. She is still within reach — I will use some of those phone-call minutes to call her — but it is a breaking of ties. When she left, she bought a round-trip ticket; but, her condo is for sale and all her possessions reside elsewhere. I decided to take a hiatus, and I will go on with the "L's" another day.

If I thought keeping a steno pad with your daily list of to-dos was a way to preserve memories, an even better source is an out-of-date address book. I'm thinking that once I have transcribed all the old pages, I will save them, along with the calendars and the notepads. What a challenge for future generations: to conjecture who these people were and what they meant to me. They'll never even be able to imagine the many long, complicated, rewarding relationships of this twentieth-century lady named Phyllis Greene.

As It Was in the Beginning

The first thing I do each morning — and the last thing I do each night — is run through a checklist in my mind and heart. It is the list of my children and their children — those to whom they are married, those to whom they are about to be married, those to whom they were once married — and the grandchildren, and where they all are, what they are doing, and if they are happy or if they are facing challenges. I almost cannot believe how much I love each one, for the total amount of that love seems too much for one woman to hold onto. Rather, it holds onto me, and holds me up. In the end, it is this sense of family that helps keep us young. This is not just my perception, but what readers of *Moonglow* said over and over and over: my children and grandchildren have been such great support; I could not have managed without them; they help with the checkbook; they put up the screens; they take me on errands; they get me through the day.

At night, keeping track in my mind of the busy family is almost a sheep-counting trick. Where are they this minute? En route to some distant city to work or vacation? Out to dinner? On the phone? Taking a course? Giving a course? Who is enjoying the work that must be done? Who dreams of the next step? Who, that day, has been at ballet or volleyball, or had an English exam, or played ice hockey, or worked to cast or write a TV show, or has been in a play, or played golf, or has written a term paper, or has gone off to camp for the first time, or has flown to visit a friend for the weekend, or has looked for a summer job, or had a sleep-over party? Do any of them, I wonder, think of me, as they doze off after all their busy-ness? They must, they must, for I can feel our thoughts of one another cross in the night air, as I count my blessings for another day.

And when the morning comes, I get to think and count and remember all over again; to hope that the day ahead will see their problems solved, their outlook bright, their world secure.

Put this on the plus side of the getting-older ledger. It is the plus that cancels all the negatives. It is the hope for generations to come. As Bob loved to say, in a phrase that made it his own: "And that's what it's all about it."

About the Author

Phyllis Greene is a Phi Beta Kappa graduate of Wellesley College. She has had a lifelong involvement in her community, having served as chairman of the board of Franklin University, the United Community Council, and the Columbus Metropolitan Airport and Aviation Commission. In 2001, she was the recipient of the Columbus Metropolitan Library's Julian Sinclair Smith Celebration of Learning Award. She is the mother of three and the grandmother of eight. She lives in Columbus, Ohio.

Phyllis Greene can be reached at:
6956 East Broad Street # 173
Columbus, Ohio 43213
or wedewede@aol.com
or www.familyhistories.com